Modified Essay Questions
for the MRCGP Examination

Modified Essay Questions for the MRCGP Examination

Edited by
T. S. MURRAY

PhD, FRCP, FRCGP, DRCOG
Senior Lecturer in General Practice, University of Glasgow.
West of Scotland Adviser in General Practice.
Examiner RCGP

Foreword by
J.G.R. HOWIE

James McKenzie Professor of General Practice
University of Edinburgh

BLACKWELL SCIENTIFIC PUBLICATIONS
Oxford London Edinburgh
Boston Palo Alto Melbourne

© 1986 by
Blackwell Scientific Publications
Editorial offices:
Osney Mead, Oxford OX2 0EL
25 John Street, London WC1N 2BL
23 Ainslie Place, Edinburgh EH3 6AJ
3 Cambridge Center, Cambridge
  Massachusetts 02142, USA
54 University Street, Carlton
  Victoria 3053, Australia

Other Editorial Offices:
Librairie Arnette SA
2, rue Casimir-Delavigne
75006 Paris
France

Blackwell Wissenschafts-Verlag
Meinekestrasse 4
D-1000 Berlin 15
Germany

Blackwell MZV
Feldgasse 13
A-1238 Wien
Austria

First published 1986
Reprinted 1987, 1992

Photoset by Enset (Phototypesetting),
Midsomer Norton, Bath, Avon
and printed and bound in
Great Britain by
Billing and Sons Ltd
Worcester

DISTRIBUTORS

Marston Book Services Ltd
PO Box 87
Oxford OX2 0DT
(*Orders*: Tel: 0865 791155
    Fax: 0865 791927
    Telex: 837515)

USA
  Blackwell Scientific Publications, Inc.
  3 Cambridge Center
  Cambridge, MA 02142
  (*Orders*: Tel: 800 759-6102
       617 225-0401)

Canada
  Times Mirror Professional Publishing, ▌
  5240 Finch Avenue East
  Scarborough, Ontario M1S 5A2
  (*Orders*: Tel: 800 268-4178
       416 298-1588)

Australia
  Blackwell Scientific Publications
  (Australia) Pty Ltd
  54 University Street
  Carlton, Victoria 3053
  (*Orders*: Tel: 03 347-0300)

British Library
Cataloguing in Publication Data

Modified essay questions for the
MRCGP examination.
    1. Family medicine—Problems,
    exercises, etc.
    I. Murray, T.S.   II. Royal College of
    General Practitioners
    610′.76   RC58

ISBN 0–632–01457–1

Contents

List of Contributors
All are currently examiners for the MRCGP

J. C O H E N MSc, BS, FRCGP, DipSoc, *Senior Lecturer in General Practice, Middlesex Hospital Medical School and General Practitioner, London*

A. P. L E W I S MA, MB BChir, DCH, DRCOG, MRCGP, *General Practitioner, Hayle, Cornwall*

J. F. M c K E L L I C A N MB, ChB, MRCGP, *Honorary Tutor, Department of General Practice, University of Dundee and General Practitioner, Dundee*

T. S. M U R R A Y PhD, FRCP, FRCGP, DRCOG, *Senior Lecturer in General Practice, University of Glasgow. West of Scotland Adviser in General Practice*

A. R E E D MB, BS, DRCOG, FRCGP, *Associate Regional Adviser, Northern Region and General Practitioner, Penrith, Cumbria*

G. B. T A Y L O R MB, BS, MRCGP, DRCOG, *General Practitioner, Guide Post Health Centre, Northumberland. Associate Regional Adviser, Postgraduate Institute, Newcastle upon Tyne*

I. W. T A Y L O R MB, ChB, MRCGP, DRCOG, *General Practitioner, Portsoy, Banffshire*

T. L. V E N A B L E S MA, MB, BChir, MRCP, FRCGP, *Principal in General Practice, Calverton, Nottinghamshire. Lecturer in General Practice, University of Nottingham*

J. W A L K E R DFC, MB, ChB, FRCGP, *Associate Adviser in General Practice, Ayrshire and General Practitioner, Ayr*

Foreword

Examinations have advantages and disadvantages. By their presence they define the territory of a subject and in turn determine the course of both training and learning. The closer examinations get to being valid measures of the attainment of true priorities of knowledge, skill and attitudes the more they will be accepted as a useful part of a discipline's portfolio of activities. General practice medicine has worked hard over a short period of time to outline, for those who work in it, what is needed in knowledge and under standing, and it has been remarkably successful.

The examination for membership of its Royal College has achieved an impressive degree of acceptance, especially considering the fact that passing it is not a required criterion for entry to Principal status.

At the same time, many who teach trainees are genuinely anxious that passing the examination is now seen as the purpose of vocational training and rightly feel concern that this is a wrong priority. At present the best-of-both worlds solution is to be able to combine the real educational potential of the various parts of the membership examination with a measure of sensible training in the techniques of presenting oneself to the examiners to ones best advantage. The Modified Essay Question (MEQ) technique has been developed by the RCGP examiners to the point where it is now widely recognized as being both a fair assessment of the process of clinical decision making and also a splendid educational facility for students at all stages of undergraduate and postgraduate education.

This short book presents 20 MEQs prepared and annotated by a team of general practitioners with many years experience of examining in the MRCGP. The editor and the originator of the idea is Dr Stuart Murray, an experienced University general practice teacher, also a College examiner and now a Regional Adviser in the West of Scotland area. Together the team have assembled a menu which will give student, teacher and candidate a splendidly concise and concentrated source of material relevant to thinking about, teaching about and writing about the job of being a family doctor. No doubt

the model answers presented may change as time progresses, but
the usefulness of the approach will surely last.

J.G.R. Howie

Preface

The first examination for membership of the Royal College of General Practitioners was held in November 1965 when five candidates sat the examination. Council decided in 1968 that only candidates who had passed the examination would be admitted for membership.

The first compulsory examination held in November 1968 attracted 32 candidates and by 1971 the annual total exceeded 163. Within 4 years this had risen to an annual total of 400 and within a further 4 years to over 1200. At present over 1600 candidates are examined for the MRCGP each year.

Preparation for the examination has become an important part of any candidate's curriculum with a constant demand for material which is related to the examination.

There are a number of books on the MCQ, and the PTQ part of the written is a well known form of examination.

The MEQ is particular to the MRCGP and is an evolving case history in a general practice setting. The candidate responds in the light of information available and the case develops. The questions tend to be open ended. The inter-relationship between behaviour and clinical medicine is dealt with in some detail with the decision making processes, which lead to some of the answers, being tested. The problems can have a clinical base but they also test problem solving, decision making and attitudes in addition to factual knowledge.

The MEQ is a real patient situation which presents the candidate with a clinical test which requires thought and experience. Trainees find this part of the written examination most difficult and they will benefit from working through the problems in the book.

All nine contributors are presently examiners for the MRCGP. Each has produced two problems with the editor producing four.

All the examiners are extremely grateful to their colleagues who helped with testing the MEQs, formulating the responses and preparing the marking schedules.

Chapter 1
The Work of a General Practitioner

The name general practitioner means many things to a great number of people but the definition which is most commonly used is in the RCGP *The Future General Practitioner.**

A description of the work of the general practitioner

The general practitioner is a licensed medical graduate who gives personal, primary and continuing care to individuals, families and a practice population, irrespective of age, sex and illness. It is the synthesis of these functions which is unique. He will attend his patients in his consulting room and in their home and sometimes in a clinic or a hospital. His aim is to make early diagnoses. He will include and integrate physical, psychological and social factors in his considerations about health and illness. This will be expressed in the care of his patients. He will make an initial decision about every problem which is presented to him as a doctor. He will undertake the continuing management of his patients with chronic, recurrent or terminal illness. Prolonged contact means that he can use repeated opportunities to gather information at a pace appropriate to each patient and build up a relationship of trust which he can use professionally. He will practice in cooperation with other colleagues, medical and non-medical. He will know how and when to intervene through treatment, prevention and education to promote the health of his patients and their families. He will recognize that he also has a professional responsibility to the community.

Educational aims

From this broad description of the general practitioner are derived the following educational aims which should be attained by the time a doctor enters independent practice. Many aims are important for

*Royal College of General Practitioners (1969) The educational needs of the future general practitioner. *J. roy. Coll. gen. Practit.*, **18**, 358.

all doctors. They are arranged in three groups: knowledge; skills; attitudes. All three groups are important in general practice.

At the conclusion of the vocational training programme, the doctor should be able to demonstrate:

Knowledge
1 That he has sufficient knowledge of disease processes, particularly of common diseases, chronic diseases and those which endanger life or have serious complications or consequences.
2 That he understands the opportunities, methods and limitations of prevention, early diagnosis and management in the setting of general practice.
3 His understanding of the way in which interpersonal relationships within the family can cause health problems or alter their presentation, course and management, just as illness can influence family relationships.
4 An understanding of the social and environmental circumstances of his patients and how they may affect a relationship between health and illness.
5 His knowledge and appropriate use of the wide range of interventions available to him.
6 That he understands the ethics of his profession and their importance for the patient.
7 That he understands the basic methods of research as applied to general practice.
8 An understanding of medico-social legislation and of the impact of this on the patient.

Skills
1 How to form diagnoses which take account of physical, psychological and social factors.
2 That he understands the use of epidemiology and probability in his every day work.
3 Understanding and use of the factor 'time' as a diagnostic, therapeutic and organizational tool.
4 That he can identify persons at risk and take appropriate action.
5 That he can make relevant initial decisions about every problem presented to him as a doctor.
6 The capacity to cooperate with medical and non-medical professionals.
7 Knowledge and appropriate use of the skills of practice management.

Attitudes

1   A capacity for empathy and for forming a specific and effective relationship with patients and for developing a degree of self-understanding.

2   How his recognition of the patients as unique individuals modifies the ways in which he elicits information and makes hypotheses about the nature of the problems and their management.

3   That he understands that helping patients to solve their own problems is a fundamental therapeutic activity.

4   That he recognizes that he can make a professional contribution to the wider community.

5   That he is willing and able critically to evaluate his own work.

6   That he recognizes his own need for continuing education and critical reading of medical information.

This in-depth analysis forms the basis of the Leeuwenhurst Statement which was formulated in 1974.

The MEQ tests many aspects of a general practitioner's work, especially those involving the skills and attitudes previously mentioned.

Chapter 2
The MRCGP Examination

The MRCGP examination at present has three written papers each giving an equal proportion of the written marks. These are Multiple Choice Questions, a Modified Essay Question and three Practice Topic Questions.

The Multiple Choice Paper consists of 60 questions each of which has five true/false stems with the 60 questions being divided in a representative way according to their importance in general practice. Two hours are allowed for this.

The Modified Essay Question (MEQ) will be the subject of a later section.

The Practice Topic Question (PTQ) consists of three questions which have to be completed in two hours. This can include clinical topics, areas of current interest in general practice or management situations.

The purpose of any professional examination is to assess the extent to which the specific educational objectives related to the job definition have been achieved. If it is to be effective the examination must be valid and reliable: a great deal of work has gone into the MRCGP to achieve this. When educational objectives are categorized they are normally concerned with three specific areas: knowledge, the cognitive domain; skills, the psychomotor domain; attitudes, the affective domain.

At present the MRCGP examination consists of the assessment of the knowledge and level of competence appropriate to the general practitioner on completion of his vocational training. The multiple choice tests mainly in the cognitive domain whereas the MEQ and PTQ can test all three areas.

Around 85% of candidates are called for two oral examinations each of which is conducted by two examiners who are unaware of the candidate's marks in the written papers. Oral 1 is based on the candidate's log diary and deals with practice organization and patients noted in the log diary. Oral 2 is the problem solving oral when problems are presented to the candidate by the examiners.

Each of the five parts of the examination provide 20% of the final mark. At present the trainee pass rate for the examination is around 70%.

Chapter 3
Modified Essay Question

The Modified Essay Paper assesses aspects of interpretation, problem solving, behaviour and attitude. This is carried out when a candidate works through a clinical problem. The Modified Essay Question (MEQ) is an original development of Royal College of General Practitioners,* of the patient management questionnaire format widely used in undergraduate and postgraduate medical education both at home and overseas.

The MEQ paper is presented in the form of a booklet. Each page presents a separate problem which must be answered before proceeding to the next page. A specific set of instructions which accompany each problem is given later. Further information is then divulged and new problems are posed as the case develops. The case is real and this open-ended approach allows the exploration of areas affecting the candidate's clinical decision making. Recall of clinical material with a behavioural pattern in a defined period of time, with the influences of factors both in patient and doctor play a part in this development. The MEQ now demands considerable understanding of the behavioural approach in the consultation if it is to be tackled successfully.

The questions tend to be composed in a way which forces the generation of a range of options with the candidates considering the advantages and disadvantages of each before making a decision. Selective use of information can be more important than opting for the one correct answer.

The MEQ has been used to test skills of information gathering via history taking, examination and the use of investigations and procedures. It has also been used for hypothesis formation and testing, evaluation of collected matter, definitions of a problem given from a physical, social and psychological viewpoint. It can also test the skills of decision making, and of communicating with colleagues, patients and relatives. The preparation of management plans taking into account the patient's problem and those within the community are important areas of a general practitioner's work. Continuity of

*Hodgkin G.K.H. & Knox J.D.E. (1975) *Problem Centred Learning.* Churchill Livingstone, Edinburgh and London.

care with appropriate use of the practice team and plans for antici-patory care are also areas which can be part of an MEQ and which reflect modern general practice.

From the large number of areas tested by the MEQ its value as a teaching tool is obvious. When used for teaching the MEQ is completed individually, then the teaching points and answers are discussed in a group. This allows the experienced doctor the oppor-tunity to explain the respective weighting of the marking schedule. In the MEQ the trainee usually gives a higher priority than the experienced doctor to the knowledge component.

When used for assessment the MEQ is examiner weighted and a short commentary will be given at the end of each MEQ to bring out the important points and why the marking schedule was so decided.

The MEQ is usually produced by one person. It is then given to a small number of colleagues who comment on the question and give their criticisms. A group then meet and formulate the answers, develop a marking schedule and give respective ratings to the different parts. An MEQ takes between $1\frac{1}{4}-1\frac{3}{4}$ hours and the time constraint is an important part of the problem as it simulates the real situation in general practice. The two main disadvantages of the MEQ format are that the candidates may gain some advantage by reading through the paper before they begin. Secondly they may answer the question in terms of what they believe the Examiner wishes to hear rather than what they actually do.

When a problem is answered it is important to remember that actual factual knowledge may be given a lower priority than decision making and problem solving skills. It is important that when marking a paper after completing the MEQ one does so as accurately as possible against the marking schedule; an alternative suggestion may be that someone else does it. One should only complete one question at a time and answers are best given in short headings and short notes.

Typical set of instructions

1   There are (actual number inserted) questions in this MEQ paper.

2   Answers should be brief, legible and concise. Total time allowed is (actual time inserted).

3   Answers should be written in the space provided. If more room is required use the reverse side of the question sheet.

4   In those questions where a definite number of answers are asked

for do not give more answers than are requested (the extra answers will not be marked).

5   You are advised not to alter your answers after completing the whole MEQ and not to look through the book before you start. This may distort your natural assessment of the case and cause you to lose marks.

6   The MEQ is a test of your practical approach to a developing general practice problem and as such you gain more marks for your management of the problem than for your pure factual knowledge.

7   The available marks vary between one question and another; you are advised to work steadily through and not delay too long on any one question.

8   Each page of the MEQ is marked independently. You should therefore answer each question specifically, even if this answer involves repetition of part of an earlier answer. [This, of course, is only true in the actual MRCGP where the marking of each page is carried out by a different examiner.]

The Questions

The questions prepared by the nine contributors cover vast areas of general practice: from very young patients to the very old, families, new patients and many other problematical areas. There is little overlap between questions thus indicating the vast breadth of general practice.

Many of the situations presented are extremely difficult and to formulate one correct response is impossible. The examiner wishes to see a range of options with an explanation as to why the candidate has followed one particular line. Each examiner with his validating colleagues has his own style and the Editor has made few alterations in the presentations and answers. The MEQ in each MRCGP examination is produced by different examiners and the breadth of experience given in the book will be valuable when the candidate actually sits the examination.

In the actual examination each page carries a maximum of 45 marks with a percentage being worked out by computer when the marks are collated. This system would be complicated in this book and the trusted system out of 100 is the easiest to follow. To have given ½ and ¼ marks would have been extremely complex but remember that with a total of 45 for each page one mark can be given for each relevant point. This emphasizes the detail each answer is given in. The larger marking (out of 45) also gives an opportunity for discretionary marking when the candidate mentions a reasonable point which the examiners had not considered. The candidate should also note that the weighting varies in different parts of the question.

In this publication, the questions have been run on from one another for ease of presentation and the candidate is advised to answer each question individually. This is obviously difficult in the present format but TRY NOT TO LOOK AHEAD. In the MRCGP examination each group of questions (indicated in this book by lines between the questions) is on a separate page. Each case is divided and a different examiner will mark each page (or clearly marked group of questions in this book). *Remember* that the examiner will not know what you wrote on a previous page so if a point needs to be repeated then *repeat it*.

Case 1

1½ hours

Your first patient on a Monday morning surgery, a Mrs Robinson, is new to the practice.

1.1 What main points would you like to discuss with her at this consultation?

You discover that she is 50 years old, married with two grown up children and one child aged 12 still at home. Her husband used to be a draughtsman but is now unemployed. The 12 year old, William, was brain damaged at birth and now takes phenobarbitone to control fits.

1.2 What main areas would you like to discuss with her at this stage?

1.3 What further agencies would you involve and why?

Mrs Robinson tells you that one of William's main problems is bed-wetting.

1.4 How would you manage this?

Two months later your health visitor stops you in the corridor of the Health Centre and tells you that she is worried about the Robinson family. She has noticed on a recent home visit that the house is very dirty and that Mrs Robinson seems unusually unkempt.

1.5 What are the possible reasons for this?

1.6 What strategies are open to you for dealing with this situation?

You see Mrs Robinson and decide that not only is she severely depressed but is also suicidal, yet refuses to have any treatment.

1.7 What options are open to you in dealing with this situation?

You are now more than halfway through the problem

You decide, after consultation with the local psychiatrist, to admit
Mrs Robinson to the local psychiatric hospital under a section. The
next morning you are rung at home at 8.15 am by a man who says he
is a solicitor acting for Mrs Robinson. He says that she has consulted
him, telling him that she is being held in the hospital against her
will.

1.8 How could you deal with this situation?

Mrs Robinson is discharged from the hospital three weeks later
apparently somewhat improved. She is taking amitryptiline
(Tryptizol) 75 mg at night. Two days later you receive a frantic
phone call during morning surgery from Mr Robinson. He tells you
that he has found his wife lying unconscious on the front room floor.

1.9 What immediate advice would you offer on the phone?

1.10 What subsequent action would you take?

You arrange for Mrs Robinson to be admitted to the local intensive
care unit. Later that day the houseman calls you to tell you that Mrs
Robinson developed an arrhythmia which they had not been able to
control and that she had died.

**1.11 What problem do you anticipate in the future with this
family?**

**1.12 Outline the strategies open to you in dealing with the
family.**

You feel very upset that despite all the care and attention that had
been given to Mrs Robinson she still killed herself.

**1.13 What strategies are open to you in dealing with your own
emotions over this?**

Case 2

1½ hours

Mrs Richardson is a 32-year-old lady who married for the second time two years ago. She was delivered of a healthy baby boy, James, five months previously after a normal pregnancy. She has two girls, aged seven and five, from her previous marriage, but they now live with their father.

She telephones you at 10.00 pm one night, telling you that James has been passing bright blood in his stools for the past 24 hours, though does not appear to have been distressed.

2.1 Outline your management, giving reasons for your actions.

James seems well and you can find nothing abnormal on physical examination and so you decide to do nothing except see James in the morning. There is no further bleeding and so you take no further action. You personally see nothing more of James until he is aged 15 months, when his mother brings him to the surgery complaining that he will not sleep.

2.2 List the main reasons that might explain this behaviour.

2.3 What options are open to you in his management?

Mrs Richardson brings James back to see you in three weeks saying that he is still sleeping badly. She tells you that a friend of hers had lent her some sleeping medicine which she had given James with good effect, allowing the family the first quiet night for weeks. She asks you to prescribe some for James.

2.4 How might you respond to this request?

2.5 What action would you take and why?

Mrs Richardson seems reluctant to take your advice. You do not see her in the surgery for a year. This time she tells you that James always has a runny nose, is snuffly, and tends to snore when he does sleep.

2.6 List the main causes for these symptoms.

2.7 Outline your management.

Mrs Richardson replies that she had another (different) friend whose child had similar symptoms which were cured by tonsillectomy. She asks you to refer James for tonsillectomy.

2.8 What main points would you like to discuss with her?

You are now more than halfway through the problem

You are on call one Saturday a few weeks later when Mrs Richardson rings you at home. Apparently her two daughters were supposed to have spent their usual weekend with her but have failed to arrive. She is particularly worried as her ex-husband had seemed under some strain recently and she had noticed some bruises on one of the girls at their last visit.

2.9 What options are open to you in managing this situation?

2.10 Which would you favour and why?

The family move away shortly after, but move back into your area when James is aged 11 and re-register on your list. Mrs Richardson rings asking for a visit for James. He has a painful right knee and is not very well. You find that he has a temperature of 38 deg., his right knee is painful on active and passive movement and there seems to be a mild effusion. There are no other joint signs.

2.11 What are the main differential diagnoses?

2.12 What options are open to you in his management?

2.13 Which would you favour and why?

After discussion of the problem with the local paediatrician, James is admitted to the local hospital. This is his first hospital admission, and he is clearly very nervous about it. The next day you are rung by a member of the local branch of the National Association for the

Welfare of Children in Hospital. She tells you that she was concerned at the distress James showed on admission and asks to attend a team meeting in your Health Centre to discuss ways in which children might be prepared for admission to hospital.

2.14 What areas might be covered at this meeting?

James is discharged from hospital with a diagnosis of juvenile chronic rheumatoid arthritis (ankylosing spondylitis type).

2.15 What points would you want to discuss with the Richardsons at your next meeting with them?

Case 3

1¼ hours

Mr C, aged 52, and Mrs C, aged 48 years, have been patients in the practice for many years. They live in a council house, and have 3 married daughters nearby. Without warning, Mr C suffers a CVA with L hemiplegia. He is lucid, articulate, and continent.
You visit him within an hour of the onset.

3.1 What factors would determine your plan of management?

3.2 What would you tell Mr and Mrs C regarding prognosis?

After several weeks of physiotherapy, Mr C's hemiparesis remains complete, and he has developed severe pain in the L leg at night.

3.3 What causes of the pain would you consider?

He has what appear to have been 2 grand mal seizures at night, and Mrs C is unable to sleep.

3.4 What are your options in dealing with this situation?

Mr C settles down, and attends a Day Centre twice a week. He is very demanding and Mrs C shows signs of strain. She tells you she has bouts of perspiration, and frequency of bowel and bladder. There is apparent weight loss.

3.5 What causes of her condition would you consider at this time?

3.6 How would you confirm or refute them?

You have several investigations pending for Mrs C, when you are called at night because she has severe abdominal pain. This has gone when you arrive, and on examination you find only slight tenderness in the R flank.

3.7 Do you consider she warrants further investigations at this stage? If so, what?

You are now more than halfway through the problem

Mrs C's daughter says she thinks her mother is trying to involve her in the care of her father. She has 3 young children and cannot give any more time.

3.8 What is your response to her?

Mrs C has a further attack next day, and you find her with signs of intestinal obstruction. She is admitted to hospital, where she is found to have carcinoma of ascending colon with spread into liver. She is sent home to her daughter, who is already caring for Mr C. Both parents think Mrs C is cured.

3.9 What is your reaction to Mrs C's discharge from hospital with an optimistic outlook?

3.10 What options do you now have, and which do you favour?

Mrs C dies quietly in bed overnight. You find Mr C withdrawn and uncooperative. He will only speak to his young grandchildren.

3.11 What do you think is behind Mr C's behaviour? Indicate its likely progress.

Case 4

1¼ hours

Mr and Mrs S lost their only child (aged 17 years) as a result of Hodgkin's Disease. They are now in their mid-sixties. Mr S has recurrent duodenal ulcer symptoms, but refuses investigation. Mrs S has taken sleeping pills since her daughter's death.

4.1 What management choices are available to you in dealing with his recurrent acute dyspepsia? Which do you favour, and why?

4.2 What are your views of Mrs S and her night sedation? What advantages/disadvantages do you see in broaching the subject with her?

Mr S consults you because of indigestion and tells you his wife is drinking (whisky) heavily, often together with her Nitrazepam. He thinks you should 'do something' about this.

4.3 What choices of reply would you consider?

4.4 Which would you favour, and why?

Mrs S calls, saying her husband had told her you wanted to see her about her drinking habits.

4.5 What responses are available to you and which do you consider most appropriate?

You are now halfway through the problem

Mr S develops L homonymous hemianopia, and asks if this event will affect his driving licence. He admits to having two short instances of loss of consciousness in the past month.

4.6 What is your reply?

4.7 What other implication do you see in his information?

4.8 What action, if any, do you consider you should take?

A year later, Mr S has a CVA with sensory aphasia, but no loss of motor function. He is unable to understand when spoken to, and gives unintelligible replies.

4.9 What courses of action are open to you, and which would you favour?

_____

Three weeks later, Mrs S phones at 7.00 am to tell you her husband has been vomiting all night and is apparently in pain.

4.10 On your way to the patient, what possibilities would occur to you as to the cause of this event?

_____

On arrival at Mr S's house, you find the patient collapsed and evidence of considerable haematemesis. You have him admitted to hospital where he is found to have a perforated duodenal ulcer. He seems to make progress after repair, but suddenly dies on 2nd post-operative day. The hospital asks you to inform his wife and seek permission for a post-mortem examination.

4.11 What is your reaction to this request?

4.12 What options do you have for dealing with it, which do you choose and why?

4.13 How do you see your role with regard to Mrs S in the near future? Specify her likely problems and your approach to them.

Case 5

1¾ hours

Your first patient in Monday morning surgery states that she overheard a stranger discussing her daughter's miscarriage with the husband of one of your receptionists.

    5.1 What do you say to the patient?

    5.2 What do you do?

On confrontation your receptionist states that the subject of the discussion, namely the girl who miscarried, had been stealing the thoughts of your receptionist.

    5.3 What further aspects of the history would you feel you have to explore bearing in mind you are her doctor as well as her employer?

A consultant opinion states 'I believe your receptionist has schizophrenia'.

    5.4 What are your obligations in relation to employment in this case?

    5.5 What is the drug therapy likely to be in this case?

Four weeks later your receptionist phones you at home when you are not on duty to tell you she thinks her husband has had a stroke and could you come right away?

    5.6 What do you do?

You are now halfway through the problem

Having examined your patient (William) you find he is aphasic and has a dense right sided hemiparesis and a homonymous hemianopia. His wife pleads with you to admit him to the district general hospital.

    5.7 Write your admission letter below.

18

Whilst in hospital William remains doubly incontinent and dysphasic. His wife tells you he is being discharged in three days and wonders what her problems are likely to be.

5.8 What problems do you foresee for both?

_____

William's improvement is very slow.

5.9 What are the long term stresses likely to be in this household?

_____

After six months there is another flare up of Marjorie's schizophrenia.

5.10 What are the possible causes for this?

5.11 What can you do?

_____

You are managing both patients at home.

5.12 What other forms of support can you make use of in this situation?

Case 6

1½ hours

Elizabeth Vernon is 76 years old and lives in a modern council bungalow with her 79-year-old husband. Twelve years ago she had a lobectomy for bronchiectasis. On a home visit at her request she tells you she has been more short of breath recently.

6.1 What other aspects of the history would you wish to elucidate?

On examination she has widespread wheezing with a prolonged expiratory phase.

6.2 What are the four most likely diagnoses. List in order of preference.

Mrs Vernon seems somewhat upset and depressed during your consultation.

6.3 What might be the possible environmental causes for this?

It transpires that her additional worry is her husband who has been wandering at night around the house and she isn't sleeping as a result of this.

6.4 What is your management plan?

A detailed examination reveals him to be a moderately demented old man who appears well-nourished, not clinically anaemic and nothing abnormal is found in his urine.

6.5 What investigations would it be reasonable to carry out at this stage?

You are now halfway through the problem

The following day Mrs Vernon's daughter telephones you to ask what you propose to do about her mother's situation since she lives five miles away and is therefore unable to help.

6.6 What do you tell her?

The situation gradually deteriorates at home over the next six months. The main problem being the worsening dementia of Mr Vernon.

6.7 What options have you for helping the situation?

While in the local geriatric unit it is discovered that Mr Vernon has maturity onset diabetes mellitus.

6.8 What problems do you forsee when discharge home is imminent?

6.9 What would your management plan be for Mr Vernon providing he was fit to remain at home?

Bearing in mind that Mrs Vernon will carry out much of the routine management,

6.10 what specific advice would you give Mrs Vernon about looking after her diabetic husband?

Case 7
1¾ *hours*

Mrs Cassidy had an iron deficiency anaemia fifteen years ago which responded well to therapy. She is now aged 55 and one month ago consulted your partner with tiredness and lassitude. Only one line is recorded in the notes stating that she was given an iron preparation and diazepam. She consults you asking for a repeat prescription.

7.1 How do you handle this situation?

7.2 What do you say to your partner?

You decide to check her blood. You repeat the prescription and arrange to see her in one week. The laboratory phone you in the late afternoon to say that the Hb is 11.9 G% with a film suggestive of chronic granulocytic leukaemia.

7.3 How would you handle this situation?

You revisit Mrs Cassidy to say that you have arranged a hospital admission for the following day. You inform her about this and she asks 'Is there anything to worry about?'

7.4 How do you respond to this?

She then asks if she can carry on with her work in the College kitchens.

7.5 What advice do you give?

Her hospital admission confirmed the diagnosis of chronic granulocytic leukaemia. Mrs Cassidy was commenced on busulphan 4 mg daily with ferrous sulphate 200 mg TID. She has also to take allopurinol 100 mg TID. You call to see her at home and learn that she has been given no information about her illness in hospital.

7.6 How do you react to this?

7.7 What would you say to Mr and Mrs Cassidy?

_____

Mrs Cassidy made a satisfactory clinical response and returned to work. One evening Mr Cassidy and his 30-year-old son come to see you at the surgery. They ask what the future holds for Mrs Cassidy.

7.8 What would you say?

_____

They also ask for guidance on how much she should be allowed to do.

7.9 Outline your response.

You are now almost halfway through the problem

Mrs Cassidy continues to do well carrying out her work and duties at home. She has several urinary tract infections over a four year period and these respond to the appropriate antibiotic.

Mrs Cassidy consults you one evening complaining about acute pain in the middle toe of her (R) foot.

7.10 Discuss the possibilities.

7.11 How would you manage this situation?

_____

The foot pain responded to aspirin and persantin therapy. Mrs Cassidy attends you on a regular basis and when aged 62 at a routine appointment she complains of lethargy and tiredness with marked weakness in her legs. She asks you if she should give up her work.

7.12 Suggest a differential diagnosis for her symptoms.

7.13 Discuss a management plan.

_____

At her next hospital attendance the marked weakness affecting her legs is noted. Examination of the central nervous system is negative and the consultant thinks that she may be depressed. You receive a note suggesting mianserin 30 mg nocté.

7.14 How do you respond to this?

One week later Mr Cassidy calls to see you extremely worried about his wife. He feels that there is something far wrong.

7.15 What do you say to him?

_____

You decide that she requires neurological investigation and she is admitted to hospital where the diagnosis of hydrocephalus secondary to cerebral atrophy is made. When allowed home Mrs Cassidy can just get about.

7.16 Outline the management problems at this stage.

Mr Cassidy, who is aged 61 and is a storeman, suggests that he must retire as his wife requires his full-time care.

7.17 How do you respond to this?

_____

There is considerable deterioration in Mrs Cassidy's condition over the following month: she now has a virtual spastic paraplegia of her lower limbs. Her husband has insisted on retirement to look after her.

7.18 What support can Mr and Mrs Cassidy be given?

_____

Mrs Cassidy dies one week later and her husband is very upset by the death.

7.19 What are the immediate problems for Mr Cassidy?

7.20 What help can you give him?

Case 8

1¾ hours

Mr James is a 40-year-old electrician who has just joined your practice. He consults you one evening stating that he wishes to lose weight. He is 170 cm and weighs 120 kg.

8.1 What other information do you require?

8.2 How do you deal with this problem?

_____

Mr James lives with his wife in a local authority house. They have no family. You do not see him for two years when he consults you about thirst and polyuria. You test his urine and find 2% glycosuria but no ketones. You note his weight is now 122 kg and he continues to smoke 20 per day.

8.3 Outline your management plan at this stage?

_____

Mrs James calls to tell you that her husband has been drinking heavily for six months. He is now missing time at work especially at the beginning of the week.

8.4 What is the significance of this information?

8.5 What further information would you ask Mrs James?

8.6 How would you deal with the problem?

_____

Mr James comes to see you at your request. He denies that there is a problem and states that he has drastically cut his alcohol intake. He has just applied for a job as an electrician on the oil rigs and is keen to get this.

8.7 If successful how would this affect the lifestyle of Mr and Mrs James?

_____

Three months later Mr James's diabetes is well controlled on metformin 850 mg BD: he has lost 12 kg in weight and states that he feels better than he has done for years. He calls for a medical examination for the oil rigs and you find a blood pressure of 190/105 both lying and standing.

8.8 What do you say to Mr James?

8.9 What is your management plan?

You are now more than halfway through the problem

His blood pressure settles to 140/85 on atenolol 100 mg daily and you decide that he can work on the oil rigs. His working pattern is two weeks on the rigs then two weeks at home.

8.10 What are the potential problems for Mr James?

8.11 From the limited information you have about her how do you think Mrs James would cope with such an arrangement?

You do not see him for eighteen months. He consults you one evening with an itch at his (L) ankle.

8.12 How do you handle this consultation?

8.13 What are the potential problems?

Six months later Mrs James calls to tell you that her husband is again drinking to excess. He pays little attention to his diet, has gained 12 kg in weight.

8.14 What action would you take?

8.15 When Mr James calls to see you, what do you say to him?

You arrange for Mr James to attend for a further appointment at the local diabetic clinic. He is again noted to be hypertensive (BP 165/100). A diuretic is added to his current regime. Two days later Mr James calls at the surgery insisting that he sees you.

At the consultation he demands to know what the future holds for him.

8.16 How do you handle this confrontation?

8.17 Why may he be taking such an attitude?

8.18 What is his long-term outlook?

Case 9

1¾ hours

Mr John Williams aged 48 has been your patient for ten years. He consults you because of increasing breathlessness over six months. He attributes his symptoms to stopping smoking at that time.

9.1 What do you say in response to this?

9.2 What further information do you require?

9.3 What examination and tests would you carry out at this initial consultation?

You detect the murmur of aortic stenosis. He is normotensive but grossly overweight (94 kg): this he attributes to stopping smoking.

9.4 What do you say to Mr Williams?

9.5 Outline your management plan.

You arrange a cardiological opinion: he is seen by the Registrar who thinks the main problem is severe hypertension (blood pressure 200/120 with normal fundi) and obesity. E.C.G. and Chest X-ray negative. Aortic stenosis not haemodynamically significant.

9.6 Comment on the Registrar's opinion.

Mr Williams asks you exactly what is wrong with him and can he continue his work as a taxi-driver.

9.7 How do you respond to this?

Mr William's blood pressure settles without treatment and he loses 10 kg in weight. The cardiologist discharges him but asks you to re-refer him if there is any deterioration in his symptoms.

The day before one of his routine visits you receive a letter from his sister telling you that he is again smoking 20 per day.

9.8 How do you handle this situation at his next consultation?

9.9 From your experience, discuss the value of health education *re* smoking during the consultation. How might you educate about smoking?

Over the next year Mr Williams has several episodes of mild cardiac failure: this responds to a thiazide diuretic. He consults you as an emergency because of a two day history of a film over his (R) eye.

9.10 Discuss possible causes.

9.11 Outline a management plan.

You are now halfway through the problem

You now note a carotid bruit and he is commenced on aspirin. A further appointment is arranged with the cardiologist who arranges an admission for cardiac catheterization. The diagnosis of moderate aortic valve stenosis is confirmed and he is placed on the waiting list for aortic valve replacement.

9.12 Mr Williams asks you at his next appointment about the risks of cardiac surgery. How do you respond?

After listening to your opinion he informs you that a workmate died during this operation three years previously.

9.13 Why has he mentioned this?
   How do you respond?

He has an uneventful post-operative period and is discharged nine days after operation with a biological aortic valve. You are asked to visit him at the home of a lady friend. You learn from your partner that he left his wife one month before the operation.

9.14 List the problems which could result from this situation.

9.15 How do you handle the consultation?

You visit Mr Williams regularly over the next few weeks and he makes an excellent recovery. You are given several nice gifts over this time.

9.16 What is the significance of this?

9.17 Mr Williams asks you about his prognosis. How do you respond?

Mr Williams although better seems to be reluctant to return to work. He informs you that his wife has commenced divorce proceedings.

9.18 What is the likely cause of his attitude?

9.19 What health problems can divorce present?

Ten months later Mr Williams comes to see you. He is being re-admitted to hospital for a coronary angiogram. He is asymptomatic and wonders if this is necessary.

9.20 What do you say to him?

9.21 What is his future prognosis?

Case 10

1½ hours

Mary Boyle aged 33 has been a patient for 5 years. She is seen infrequently, always for self-limiting conditions. She is an unmarried secretary living with her parents in a local authority house. The family are practising Roman Catholics. She consults you one evening announcing that she is pregnant and would like you to arrange a termination.

10.1 How do you conduct this consultation?

10.2 Why do you think Mary has taken such a definite attitude about pregnancy?

Mary has had a relationship with a married man, a colleague at work, for the last six months. He has a young family, feels sorry for Mary's plight and is keen that she has an abortion.

10.3 What advice would you give Mary at this time?

10.4 What other agencies could help her?

You try to counsel Mary suggesting support from her family and the local Parish Priest. You arrange to see her in a week but the day before the consultation you receive a letter from the British Pregnancy Advisory Service in a town 200 miles away stating that a termination was carried out three days previously. She has been started on the 'pill'.

10.5 How do you react to this news?

Mary arrives for her consultation the following day. How do you conduct this?

10.6 What advice do you give her?

Eight days later you receive a Deputizing Service slip stating that Mary had been seen the night before with severe chest pain:

examination was uninformative and a diagnosis of bad gastritis and oesophagitis was made. The patient was given 100 mg pethidine i.m. and a prescription for an antacid. No follow-up arrangements were made.

10.7 What would you do?

10.8 What are the other diagnostic possibilities?

When you called to see her, you found her fairly comfortable. An E.C.G. and Chest X-ray were arranged. The latter shows an enlarged heart with a small area of opacity in the lateral part of the (R) mid-zone. You revisit and she is still dyspnoeic.

10.9 Give your management at this time.

10.10 What explanation do you give to Mary for her symptoms?

You are now more than halfway through the problem

Mary makes a good recovery in hospital. She is discharged on warfarin, frusemide and a potassium supplement. You visit her at home and she asks you exactly what has been wrong with her.

10.11 What do you say?

10.12 What is your management plan over the next few months.

Mary makes a good recovery and her therapy is gradually tailed off. She calls at the surgery four months later to inform you that she has just got engaged to an engineer who has just moved to the area. She is happy and wants to thank you for all the help you have been to her. She wonders if having a termination will reduce her chances of becoming pregnant in the future.

10.13 How do you respond to this?

Her fiancé does not know about her termination and she asks you whether she should tell him.

10.14 What do you say?

Mary tells her fiancé about the termination and he seems to accept this. They arrange their marriage six months ahead: they are keen to have a family but not in the immediate future. Mary consults you about contraceptive advice.

10.15 What do you say?

10.16 What routine checks would you like to carry out?

Mary was thrilled when she became pregnant three years later (now 39) but unfortunately had an incomplete abortion at 12 weeks followed by a dilatation and curettage.

10.17 What support could she be given at this time?

10.18 Outline the long term problems which she may have?

Case 11

1½ hours

Mrs Jamieson, the wife of a 32-year-old dentist, telephones you at 8.30 on a Monday morning just before you are due to start surgery saying that her husband has been vomiting all night and that she would like you to call.

11.1 What factors would influence you in your response to this request?

When you visit you find that he is pale and ill and gives a history of central chest pain which has lasted for some four hours. Physical examination reveals a gallop rhythm, a blood pressure of 110/84 and a regular pulse with a rate of 104 per minute. You diagnose probable myocardial infarction.

11.2 What factors should you consider when deciding between home and hospital care?

You decide to admit him to hospital where he is found to have had a massive anterior myocardial infarction. He has a persistent supraventricular tachycardia with runs of ventricular tachycardia and remains in the coronary care unit for three days. His wife asks you to visit him in hospital because he wishes to talk with you.

11.3 What are the areas that he might want to explore with you at this stage?

After a week in hospital he is discharged home on disopyramide. He is obviously very tense and frightened and moves about his house slowly. He has a pulse rate of 88 per minute and no abnormal physical signs.

11.4 What problems do you now face in your management?

Two weeks after his discharge a local consultant cardiologist telephones you to say that he is a friend of your patient and that he would like to assess him with a view to angiography in view of the patient's age.

11.5 What factors would you take into consideration when responding to this request?

You are now more than halfway through the problem

Three months later Mr Jamieson is still very tense and reluctant to return to work saying that he is sure that stress has contributed to his illness. He is having nightmares about the coronary care unit and has become obsessional about his weight and his eating habits.

11.6 What lines of management might be appropriate at this stage?

Two months later his wife attends with a sore throat. When leaving the consulting room she pauses at the door and asks 'Are there any tablets you can give my husband to pep up his sex drive?'

11.7 How could you respond to this?

Mr and Mrs Jamieson have four children. Richard 8, John 6, Christopher 4, and Jenny aged 2. Mr Jamieson's mother died at the age of 48 from a myocardial infarction. A year after Mr Jamieson's infarction has taken place he and his wife ask you what the implications are for the children in view of the fact that their father has had a heart attack at such a young age.

11.8 What factors would you discuss with them?

Eighteen months after his first infarction Mr Jamieson dies suddenly on Christmas Eve.

11.9 What problems will you now face in dealing with the rest of the family subsequently?

Case 12

1½ hours

Mrs Robertson is a 57-year-old farmer's wife who has two married daughters. She requests to be transferred to your list from that of a neighbouring doctor. There has not been a recent change of address.

12.1 What are the possible reasons for such a request?

_____

You agree to take her on as a patient and she attends to ask for a repeat prescription for her medication for longstanding rheumatoid arthritis.

12.2 What areas might you explore with her at this consultation?

_____

Three months later Mrs Robertson telephones during evening surgery to request a visit because of worsening arthritis. On attending her you find her to have a hot, red, swollen left knee joint. She requests immediate private specialist advice.

12.3 What are the possible reasons for her behaviour?

_____

She is admitted to a private hospital under a consultant rheumatologist's care and is found to have a septic arthritis. After three weeks in hospital she remains ill with a persistent septic arthritis of both knees and of her left elbow. Her husband attends your surgery and is clearly unhappy about the course of his wife's illness and its treatment. He asks your advice about the best plan of action.

12.4 What lines are now open to you? List the advantages and disadvantages of each.

_____

She is transferred to a National Health Service hospital under the care of a different consultant where she is found to have a septic focus in her thoracic spine with erosion of two vertebral bodies. She deteriorates rapidly and her husband requests that she be transferred home so that she may die in familiar surroundings.

12.5 What factors would influence your response to this request?

You are now more than halfway through the problem

After a long and stormy illness including a major spinal operation Mrs Robertson eventually recovers and is transferred home. She has residual tinnitus caused by the powerful antibiotics which she has received. On discharge from hospital she tells you that she wishes to sue the rheumatologist who first attended her.

12.6 How might you cope with this situation?

One month after his wife's discharge from hospital Mr Robertson attends with a story of sleep disturbance, anorexia and loss of concentration. He presents with a picture of abject depression.

12.7 What areas might it be fruitful to explore with him at this consultation?

Three months after discharge from hospital Mr and Mrs Robertson decide to go on holiday to West Africa for convalescence.

12.8 What advice would you offer?

A year later Andrea Robertson, the 23-year-old married daughter of the couple who lives in another part of the country, attends your surgery and tells you that she thinks her mother and father are drinking too much.

12.9 What lines of action are open to you?

Case 13

1¼ hours

Mr James Jones, a semi-retired gardener, aged 67, married with no children, attends the surgery with a complaint of aching pain in the left hip, of a few months duration.

13.1 What further questions would you ask of the patient?

13.2 What examination would you carry out?

———————

Examination reveals that movements of the left hip are restricted. His records show that in 1975 an X-ray of cervical spine revealed minimal spondylosis.

13.3 What further investigations would you undertake, if any?

13.4 What therapy would you recommend?

———————

You prescribe Ibuprofen tablets 400 mgm t.i.d. Ten days later, you are asked to visit by his wife who is alarmed at the persistence and severity of his pain and his threat to take an overdose of his pain-killers. An X-ray report received that morning shows minimal O.A. changes in both hips with quite marked degenerative changes in the lumbar spine.

13.5 What is your next move?

You are now halfway through the problem

On arrival at the house, you find him with continuing pain in the hip and also in the right lower chest posteriorly attributed by him to a recent injury.

Chest examination revealed marked tenderness over the lower ribs, which was the only positive finding. He appeared less well, withdrawn and anxious but denied any suicidal threats.

13.6 What action would you take?

———————

Despite reassurance and sedation he becomes increasingly tired. An X-ray of his chest shows enlargement of the right hilum.

13.7 What is the differential diagnosis?

_____

Bronchial carcinoma is confirmed by subsequent hospital investigation.

13.8 How would you manage the situation?

Case 14
1½ hours

Mr Wilson and his wife, both aged 47, and their married son, Harold, aged 24, who lives with them, have been with the practice all their lives. Doctor–patient relationship has always been good.

Mr Wilson, who owns a garage in town, comes to see you apologizing jokingly because he has no symptoms and feels 'fit as a fiddle' and explains that he is planning to expand his business in a big way. He asks you to do a general medical check to reassure him that he is physically fit to take on the extra burden over the next few years.

14.1 What three lines of questioning would you pursue at this stage?

_____

You agree to undertake the examination by appointment the following day.

14.2 What form do you envisage it taking?

_____

Physical examination of Mr Wilson the following day is negative. As he is dressing he says 'Good for another thirty years then Doc?'

14.3 What do you reply?

_____

A week later during morning surgery the Casualty Officer at the Infirmary telephones to say that Mr Wilson has collapsed at his garage and had just been brought in dead to the Infirmary. He asks if you would be prepared to issue a death certificate.

14.4 How do you reply?

_____

You suspect that Mr Wilson has died from a coronary thrombosis because of the further details of the 'collapse' given to you by the Casualty Officer.

14.5 Name five 'high risk' factors in the aetiology of coronary artery disease in young men.

You are now halfway through the problem

You decide to visit Mrs Wilson after lunch and anticipate a difficult consultation.

14.6 What are the three recognized stages of the grief reaction?

_____

On a follow-up visit to Mrs Wilson three days later, the son, Harold, is present and they jointly accuse you of negligence because you had declared Mr Wilson healthy following the examination a week prior to his death. They declare their intention to report you to the 'authorities' to protect other people from your incompetence.

14.7 How do you reply?

_____

Mrs Wilson comes to the surgery a week later asking you to forgive her for being too hasty. You wonder if she may be depressed.

14.8 Name five symptoms or signs which would help support a diagnosis of depression associated with the grief reaction.

_____

Two weeks later Harold Wilson comes to the surgery complaining of chest pains on exertion and demands to see a heart specialist.

14.9 How would you handle this situation?

Case 15

1¾ hours

Mr and Mrs Patel are an Asian couple in their forties with three children from 3–13 years. Mr Patel works as a waiter in a local Indian restaurant. He comes to the surgery one evening and says he has felt very tired and weak for several months.

15.1 How would you assess the significance of this complaint?

_____

You find nothing abnormal on examination and then he reveals that the weakness occurs after attempting intercourse.

15.2 Why do you think he presented the problem as he did?

_____

You do not find it easy to help Mr Patel and ask him and his wife to attend surgery together. At the next consultation, Mrs Patel does not come but a cousin comes, she says 'as an interpreter'.

15.3 Why is this and what does it mean?

_____

Some months later Mrs Patel brings their youngest child aged 3 years and says that he always has 'coughs and colds' and occasional 'noises in the chest'. She asks for 'strong medicine' because he is keeping everyone awake at night.

15.4 How might a GP respond to her request?

_____

Ramesh is thought to have asthma and settles quite well on oral medication. Some weeks later Mr Patel telephones and asks for a second opinion as his employer has recommended him to consult a local private practitioner.

15.5 How could you deal with this problem?

You are now halfway through the problem

A few months later Mr Patel contacts you again on the telephone and asks you to see his father who has recently arrived from India.

He says his father has had diarrhoea for weeks.

15.6 What might be the cause of his complaint and how should it be managed?

_____

Investigation of Mr Patel's father reveals hookworm and he is given treatment which successfully clears his symptoms. However he appears in the surgery a month later with his son and asks for a tonic.

15.7 How would you handle this request?

_____

Some months later Sabina, the Patel's elder daughter now aged 16 years, consults at the surgery with headaches and panic feelings which she has difficulty in controlling.

15.8 What might cause these symptoms and how would you initially manage the problem?

_____

Tests reveal thyrotoxicosis and she is treated with carbimazole but she feels she is unable to take her 'O' level examinations. Mr & Mrs Patel ask for your help.

15.9 Is there anything you can do about this and does your action have any disadvantages?

_____

15.10 What do you know about the way Asian families are organized, and could you and your Primary Care Team anticipate any problems and handle them better in the future?

Case 16

1¾ hours

Harry and Gertrude Marcus live with their son Robert, aged 17 years, and daughter Tracy, aged 15 years, in a thirties semidetached suburban house. Mrs Marcus' mother aged 79 years also lives with them. In early Spring one year Mrs Marcus, now aged 44 years, comes to the surgery complaining of heavy, prolonged periods and depression.

16.1 What might be the cause of her symptoms? Outline your management.

Gertrude settles well on progesterone in the second half of the menstrual cycle. A few weeks later Harry comes to see you very upset. He says his mother-in-law is seeing things and talking to herself and really feels it is about time she went somewhere permanently.

16.2 How would you handle this request?

Grandmother's chest infection improves and with it her mental state, but Harry sees you two or three times in a few weeks complaining of indigestion. You find nothing abnormal on examination, but antacids do not appear to help.

16.3 What are your management options and what are their advantages and disadvantages?

Harry's symptoms settle on a course of cimetidine after a negative endoscopy but the same month Tracy consults because of 'terrible spots'. You can see a few acniform spots. She asks for hormone treatment 'because it helped a friend and also because I have bad periods'.

16.4 Outline what you could do to help Tracy and what you might actually do?

Much to your surprise only the following week Harry comes to the surgery with Gertrude and tells you of Robert's abnormal behaviour. He shouts, argues and locks himself in his room. They ask you to come round right away, but agree to postpone the visit till the end of the surgery.

16.5 What possible causes may there be for this problem and how could you separate them?

You are now halfway through the problem

When you arrive Robert is locked in his room and a record player is blaring noisely; conversation with Robert is impossible but Harry offers to break down the door so that you can get in and 'deal' with the situation.

16.6 Do you agree or not and what are the implications of each move you can make?

_____

Robert is thought to have been abusing soft drugs and agrees to a period of inpatient care in the local psychiatric hospital. The psychiatrist would like to offer some family therapy and asks your help and assistance. The family in their turn also come and ask you what this therapy is and what Robert's problem has to do with them.

16.7 How do you respond?

_____

Family therapy does not really succeed and after some weeks Robert leaves hospital and goes to a hostel but does not settle very well and returns home periodically and causes much friction. Late one Saturday night when you are on duty there is an emergency request for a visit to the Marcus household. The call comes from Gertrude who says that Harry and Robert are fighting and 'you must come quickly doctor or he'll kill him'. She rings off.

16.8 What could you do now and why?

_____

With the aid of neighbours and the Police the fight is ended and Harry and Robert's superficial wounds are cleaned and dressed. Harry says he's got 'to get Robert out of the house', Gertrude is crying, mother is asleep upstairs and Tracy is out. Robert says he didn't start it. You find Robert has formally left the hostel and has been staying at home or sleeping rough.

16.9 How do you handle this current situation?

_____

After years of infrequent consultation, you find on review that this family have generated about 20 consultations and 8 visits in a year.

16.10 Why should this be and what, if anything, could have been done earlier to prevent these problems arising?

Case 17
1½ hours

Thomas is a bachelor of 61 years of age, and a railway engine driver, who has been found to be suffering from cervical spondylosis, severe enough to give him temporary obstruction to cerebral blood flow on sudden neck movements. He also has peptic ulceration and mild hypertension. He has been off work for several weeks, because of his cervical spondylosis, and is now thinking of returning to work. He comes to tell you that he has to see the 'Railway Doctor', and wants to know what will happen about his work.

17.1 What do you say to him?

———————————

Thomas gets back to work and, apart from coping quite well with his work, he has a vagotomy and pyloroplasty for a haematemesis from his duodenal ulcer. For 3 years he remains quite well, until he begins to complain of dragging in his legs when walking.

The neurologist to whom you refer him is surprised that he is still working, and thinks Thomas may have had some brain stem infarct, and perhaps further cerebral ischaemic episodes.

He is at last deemed unfit to work, and given early retirement. He announces that he will be going to stay with his fiancée of many years, who has said she will look after him.

17.2 What problems do you see in the immediate period, and in the future for Thomas?

———————————

Two years later, after a myocardial infarction, he is admitted to hospital following an overdose of Ibuprofen and alcohol. The Ibuprofen had been prescribed to help his neck and back pain. He is again referred to a neurologist by the physicians, but he sends for a home visit because he has never received his neurology appointment, and you notice the address you are requested to visit is that of his fiancée, and not that on his medical record.

17.3 How do you cope with the situation?

———————————

His fiancée thinks he should be admitted again, particularly as she is

46

soon going to be admitted herself to hospital for a hysterectomy. Thomas is just sitting in a chair, looking rather down-in-the-mouth, and there is a smell of urine in the room. His fiancée, who seems to dominate him, tells you that he is often unable to get to the toilet and asks if the nurse could come in to help him.

17.4 What problems do you see arising now, and how would you cope with them?

After pressing for admission for the period while his fiancée is in hospital, and to get him assessed further neurologically, the consultant returns him to your care, with a diagnosis of brain stem vascular disease and cerebral atrophy, with a further comment, 'Perhaps you would arrange for geriatric supervision for this man now that he is within their age group'. You note he is indeed now 65.

17.5 How would you react to this request?

You are now more than halfway through the problem

The geriatrician who does the domiciliary visit is not too thrilled at the idea of Thomas being landed on his plate, especially in view of his urinary incontinence which is deemed to be due to prostatism, and suggests that now that his fiancée is home, all effort should be made to manage him in the community, even although he acknowledges he is walking with a shuffling gait now, and may be difficult.

You are awaiting a urology opinion on Thomas anyway regarding his prostate.

17.6 What agencies can you contact and how can they help to maintain Thomas in the community?

Eventually, Thomas has a transurethral prostatectomy, but is sent home with an indwelling catheter because he cannot control his bladder. You persuade the geriatrician to take him to Day Hospital twice a week, on a Tuesday and Friday, for physiotherapy and to relieve the burden at home. He has had a fair bit of discomfort from the catheter, but your nursing sister is quite happy about things.

At 5.50 pm one Friday evening, his fiancée 'phones to say he has just returned from Day Hospital in great pain from his catheter. She has 'phoned the Day Hospital to complain about him being sent home, and says the ambulance men who brought him home say he should never have been allowed home. She tells you to call that night and admit him to hospital.

17.7 How do you feel, and what can you do?

A few weeks later, the geriatrician 'phones you to say he is fed up with Thomas's fiancée interfering so much, and playing off one service against the other. He says he has heard that she has complained to the local district councillor about the lack of care given to Thomas, but no official complaint has yet been received. However, in view of this, he suggests admitting Thomas for an independent assessment in hospital as to his capabilities, as he feels he could do much more for himself.

17.8 What skills would be assessed, and by whom, and how would this admission help the situation?

Thomas is found to be continent, happy, able to manage dressing and caring for himself in every way except cooking. A case conference is called and, after discussion, it is decided that he could manage fairly well on his own at his own home with the long term possibility of admission to a residential home for the elderly, provided he remains continent. Thomas is perfectly willing to entertain the idea of a residential home, and his fiancée is called in to the case conference to be told of the decision. It is decided that as you are attending the case conference as Thomas's G.P., and know the fiancée as well, although she is not a patient of yours, you should be the spokesman for the group.

17.9 What would you say to her, and what do you think briefly would be the outcome of this?

Case 18
1½ hours

Mr Jack is an 88-year-old retired policeman who lives with his 90-year-old wife in a modern local authority house, 2½ miles from your surgery. He has a history of chronic obstructive airways disease and a previous myocardial infarction. His wife is not on your NHS list. They tend to be very independent. They have no family.

18.1 What problems are likely to arise as they get older?

_____

You are asked to visit Mr Jack at home because of an exacerbation of his chest condition. He tells you he has got dirty spit, and is having difficulty in breathing. He has a fever, is obviously dyspnoeic, and has sounds in his chest compatible with a super-imposed chest infection. His wife is hobbling around on a Zimmer, and very anxious.

18.2 Detail factors which would influence your decision whether to treat him at home or admit him.

_____

You reluctantly accept his plea that he is not bad enough for hospital, but when your assistant visits two days later, he is confronted by a neighbour who says Mr Jack ought to be in hospital and Mrs Jack cannot cope.

Your assistant manages to placate the neighbour, and comes to discuss the situation with you, having said he would have an answer tomorrow.

18.3 What do you and your assistant discuss?

_____

Having decided that admission would be appropriate, your assistant telephones the hospital, and is told that there won't be a bed for at least 2 days in Mr Jack's usual respiratory unit.

18.4 What can be done at this stage?

You are now halfway through the problem

After his discharge from hospital, you find Mr Jack alone in the house. His wife was admitted to a local authority home while he was in hospital, but was admitted from there to the local geriatric hospital as an emergency. Mr Jack is very aggrieved at his wife's 'mismanagement', and says her doctor should be struck off, as he had obviously been mismanaging her.

18.5 How do you react to this, and discuss his immediate management.

On your next visit, Mr Jack produces Mrs Jack's medical card, and says he wants you to take her on your list. He has signed the card.

18.6 What options are open to you?

You accept the wife on your list. She comes home from hospital. You find she was admitted to the geriatric department because of dehydration, and failure to eat in the local authority home. There is also a diagnosis of sideroblastic anaemia and osteoarthritis. A referral has been made to orthopaedics for consideration of right hip replacement, and the orthopaedic surgeons have agreed to do this. Mr Jack says something will have to be done also about his wife's eyesight. The hospital told them she had a cataract.

18.7 How do you feel about the management of Mrs Jack now, and what steps would you take?

The Jacks settle down with Mrs Jack waiting for her hip replacement and in the interval she has had one cataract attended to. All has settled down quite well until one evening when you are called to Mrs Jack who is in congestive cardiac failure, and has to be admitted as an emergency. Mr Jack remains at home, and the next morning when discussing the couple with your health visitor and nurse, your receptionist informs you that a neighbour of Mr Jack has just 'phoned to say that he has been coughing up blood all night and that something will have to be done for him.

18.8 What do you do?

Case 19

1½ hours

Tom and Jessie Scott, although your patients for many years, are rarely seen in the surgery. Tom, 50, is a miner whilst Jessie works part-time as a secretary for the NCB. They have a son Bill, who is 25 and has followed his father into the mines. The local papers are full of the possibility of a mining strike, when Tom presents himself at your surgery. He complains of severe gripping chest pains, which spread to his left arm and seem to be associated with exertion.

19.1 What is your differential diagnosis at this stage?

19.2 Outline your management of Tom at this consultation.

Tom is a heavy smoker, forty a day. As is the local custom he drinks large volumes of beer at weekends, but none during the week. From your history and examination you believe he may have developed angina. In view of his employment you decide to certify him unfit for work.

19.3 What do you say to Tom?

19.4 Outline the short and long term consequences of this diagnosis for Tom.

Four weeks later when the strike has become a reality, you are called to see Tom at home. You had prescribed glyceryl trinitrate and beta blockers to control his angina and initially this seemed to be successful. When you see him he is still complaining of chest pain on exertion and he looks flat and apathetic. While you are in his home you notice that Jessie has taken on a new lease of life and seems a much more outgoing woman than you remember.

19.5 Why might Tom's angina not be improving?

19.6 Give reasons for Tom and Jessie's apparent incongruities and any long term consequences you can forsee.

Tom tells you that he is being called a 'scab' by his workmates, who believe he is fabricating his symptoms to avoid picket duty. He tells you that he wants to be 'signed off' for the next week.

19.7 Outline your response to Tom.

You are now halfway through the question

Tom decides to join the strike despite your advice. Three days later you are called to see him at home late at night. Jessie tells you that he has been in police custody for a few hours charged with assaulting a Police Officer whilst on picket duty. Jessie is extremely upset and crying. Concerned neighbours are pressing you to 'give her something'.

19.8 What problems do you face at this time, and how could you deal with them?

You spend some time talking to Jessie who settles down. Tom tells you that he was merely part of the crowd when arrested. He asks if he should get a solicitor to fight his case and also asks if you would provide him with medical evidence as to his innocence.

19.9 How would you respond to these two requests, and why?

As you are leaving the house Bill angrily tells you that he is sick of having no money and that he is having to sell his own home as he can no longer afford to pay the mortgage. All this is going to change he says as he is going to do 'a bit of thieving'.

19.10 What problems do you face, and how would you manage them?

While discussing this case with your partners the next day, your senior partner declares that the strike is causing a terrible increase in work. Your other partners nod in agreement. You are however, uncertain about this.

19.11 How could you confirm or deny your partner's statement?

Case 20

1½ hours

You are called late one night to see a febrile two-year-old girl. The family are new to your list and you have no records available.

20.1 Which areas would you cover in this consultation?

_____

You discover that Tom and Jennie have moved into the area whilst Tom, who is unskilled, looks for work. They have two children, Fergus who is seven and Fiona who is two. The family have no relatives in the area and have been housed by the council on an estate usually used for 'problem families'.

20.2 What problems might this family face?

20.3 Are there any ways that you can help them?

_____

Fiona has a self-limiting upper respiratory tract infection which you treat conservatively. You lose sight of the family until you are approached by your Health Visitor one month later. She tells you that she is concerned because Fiona is 'failing to thrive'. She has asked for the mother and child to attend your surgery later that day.

20.4 What is meant by 'failing to thrive'? How could you confirm this at your initial consultation?

20.5 If the child is failing to thrive, list likely reasons why, and how you would initially investigate these possibilities as a General Practitioner.

_____

You discover that Fiona eats an extremely deficient diet. This appears to be made up of packet soups and crisps. Jennie seems totally unconcerned by this diet.

20.6 Give reasons for Jennie's attitude.

20.7 How would you manage this situation?

You are now halfway through the problem

53

Your Health Visitor agrees to monitor the family closely and the Social Services become involved to ensure adequate finance for the family. You are approached by the Social Worker who asks if she can give the family's name to a local group who provide holidays and toys for needy families.

20.8 How would you respond to this, and why?

Jennie is obviously pleased by your interest in the family and tells you with great embarrassment one day that Fergus still wets the bed.

20.9 What are the possible causes for this?

Jennie agrees to bring Fergus to see you and when you examine him he seems to have no physical abnormality.

20.10 List possible management options and their pros and cons.

Sitting thinking about this case makes you recognize that there are deficiencies in your practice organization.

20.11 How can a GP organize his practice to maximize the help he gives to socially deprived patients?

Case 1

Answers

Case 1, Answers

Your first patient on a Monday morning surgery, a Mrs Robinson, is new to the practice.

    1.1 What main points would you like to discuss with her at this consultation?

Name, address, date of birth
Significant past history
   illnesses
   pregnancies
Family history
   husband
   children
   parents
   relations
Smoking and alcohol history
Drugs
   current
   previous
Allergies
Occupation
Housing
Finances
Last cervical smear
Tet. vacc. status
Any current problems
   medical
   family
   social
Reason for attendance   8
Practice policies
How to get a visit
Repeat prescribing
Other relevant practice matters
Clearly too many questions for a Monday morning.

Concept of practice nurse delivering new patient questionnaire useful.

Much of practice matters could be imparted in practice booklet
or by receptionist or by practice nurse if she does initial
health check. $\frac{4}{12}$

_____

You discover that she is 50 years old, married with two grown up
children and one child aged 12 still at home. Her husband used to be
a draughtsman but is now unemployed. The 12 year old, William,
was brain damaged at birth and now takes phenobarbitone to control fits.

**1.2 What main areas would you like to discuss with her at this
stage?**

Problems related to William
  Medical
    are fits controlled?
    other medical problems?
    drug therapy?
    ?side effects ?best drug
  Social
    effect on family life of late child
    effect on family life of having handicapped child
    finances and allowances (unemployed)
    attendance allowance
  Schooling
    special
    normal.   8

1.3 What further agencies would you involve and why?

Probably no further agencies at this stage.
Later
  health visitor
  social services should see all disabled on their patch (legal
    obligation)
  education services
  voluntary agencies: local childrens' welfare groups
                      epilepsy association
(All with family's consent.) $\frac{4}{12}$

_____

Mrs Robinson tells you that one of William's main problems is bed-wetting.

1.4 How would you manage this?

Ask to see child in surgery
  ? primary or secondary
  ? side effects of drugs
Primary
  ? need to investigate
  full history
  ? daytime enuresis
  ? dribbles
  examine kidneys
        bladder
        urine stream
        ? neurogenic bladder
  further invest—MSU, ?IVP, ? urea and electrolytes, ?MSU
    (needs pros and cons)   6
  should probably be referred
Secondary Significant % of children of his age still wet, but
  treatment probably advisable
Methods: star chart (can he manage this?)
        enuresis alarm,
          full explanation on how to use it
        drugs, but effect of tricyclics on phenobarbitone
        health visitor
May need referral if abnormality found e.g. neurogenic
  bladder
  or reflux
  or structural abnormality   6
If no response refer either to paediatrician or child psychiatry
  or family therapy
Other aids e.g. mattress, rubbers, financial.   2
                                                  14

Two months later your health visitor stops you in the corridor of the Health Centre and tells you that she is worried about the Robinson family. She has noticed on a recent home visit that the house is very dirty and that Mrs Robinson seems unusually unkempt.

1.5 What are the possible reasons for this?

Physical
  hypothyroidism
  presenile dementia
  drug or alcohol abuse   3
Mental
  depressive illness
  psychotic illness
  non-coping behaviour   3
Social
  family discord
  marital discord
  wife battering
  economic crisis   3

1.6 What strategies are open to you for dealing with this situation?

Ask health visitor to take appointment to Mrs Robinson
Visit yourself
Ask social services to call and assess
Ask health visitor to follow up family.   3
                                                                        ____
                                                                         12

You see Mrs Robinson and decide that not only is she severely depressed but is also suicidal, yet refuses to have any treatment.

1.7 What options are open to you in dealing with this situation?

Involve husband
Spend more time counselling her in surgery
Make a longer appointment to see her next day (but real risk of
    suicide bid)
Involve health visitor
Involve social worker
Consult local psychiatrist (Domiciliary visit or urgent out-
    patient appointment)
Consider compulsory admission to psychiatric hospital
Knowledge of relevant sections important (particularly
    problems associated with their use)
Consider effects of your action on long term relationships with
    her and her family

Is section essential; is there way one can manage her at home
without admitting?
How will family with disabled child manage without her?
Consider other disadvantages of compulsory admission.
Option must really be to favour section, if necessary, on
grounds that illness is potentially reversible and risks of
staying at home are too great. 10

You decide, after consultation with the local psychiatrist, to admit
Mrs Robinson to the local psychiatric hospital under a section. The
next morning you are rung at home at 8.15 am by a man who says he
s a solicitor acting for Mrs Robinson. He says that she has consulted
him telling him that she is being held in the hospital against her will.
1.8 How could you deal with this situation?

You have no idea who this man is so no information can be
given over the phone. On the other hand the interests of
your patient are at heart and it is possible that she has been
sectioned in error; she certainly seems to have insight into
her condition now. 3
Options
Decline
Agree and release information over telephone (breach of
confidentiality)
Discuss with consultant/registrar
Suggest solicitor either writes with written consent or visits
you at your practice
Call and visit Mrs Robinson yourself and assess situation
Suggest to solicitor that a second opinion is sought
Seek advice of other bodies e.g. Medical Defence
organization, Local Medical Committee. $\frac{5}{8}$

Mrs Robinson is discharged from the hospital three weeks later
apparently somewhat improved. She is taking amitryptiline
Tryptizol) 75 mg at night. Two days later you receive a frantic
phone call during morning surgery from Mr Robinson. He tells you
hat he has found his wife lying unconscious on the front room floor.
1.9 What immediate advice would you offer on the phone?

Tell him you will visit immediately

Turn her on her side
Clear vomit, teeth from airway
Probably call ambulance now
Keep all pill bottles or other evidence of self poisoning
Get name and address and phone number.   5

1.10 What subsequent action would you take?

Visit now
Assess physical state
   level of consciousness
   pulse (arrhythmias?)
   blood pressure
   other central nervous system signs
   evidence of other medical problems e.g. diabetes, CVA,
     myocardial infarction.
Attempt to get history from husband
Find evidence of overdose and send bottles to hospital
   (remember son's phenobarbitone)
Arrange admission to hospital if not already done
Stay with patient until ambulance arrives.
Be prepared to resuscitate if necessary (need kit)
? Should go to hospital with patient. Probably not, as little you
   could do that ambulance crew can't, and would be out of
   practice.
Follow-up: ring hospital later and keep in touch with family. $\frac{7}{12}$

You arrange for Mrs Robinson to be admitted to the local intensive care unit. Later that day the houseman calls you to tell you that Mrs Robinson developed an arrhythmia which they had not been able to control and that she had died.

1.11 What problem do you anticipate in the future with this family?

Emotions
   Anger with you for not dealing adequately with problem
   guilt for not recognizing problem sooner
   bereavement stage (Murray Parkes)
     denial
     anger
     guilt
     acceptance.   5

Practical problems
     coping with disabled child
     single parent family
     increased morbidity in bereaved families
     alcohol
     suicide risk in husband.   4

1.12 Outline the strategies open to you in dealing with the family.

Visit same day
Visit once or twice after, risk of dependence
Talk about feelings he has, including his guilt and anger
Other agencies as and when appropriate
     health visitor
     social services
     local voluntary agencies
     CRUSE. $\frac{5}{\underline{14}}$

_____

You feel very upset that despite all the care and attention that had been given to Mrs Robinson she still killed herself.

1.13 What strategies are open to you in dealing with your own emotions over this?

Feelings of failure and guilt
Personal strengths and weaknesses
Talk to spouse or other close person who can help share load
Partners
Local small group
Support groups
Other agencies e.g. church.
Important not to neglect one's own feelings in tragedies such
     as this.
Openness with colleagues about one's own strengths and
     weaknesses important.   6

Commentary

The MEQ about the Robinson family explores the problems related to having a handicapped child and the examiner is looking for an answer both from the medical and social aspects. Decision making is tested in questions 1.5 and 1.6 when the doctor is told about the mother being unkempt. To obtain full marks the candidate has to consider the reasons from a physical, social and psychological aspect. Mrs Robinson's refusal of treatment tests problem solving, with the examiner looking for options and decisions as to what the candidate would so.

Question 1.8 tests aspects of confidentiality and also the doctor's attitudes towards his patient. He has again to consider options in a difficult situation. The examiner awards 14% to questions 1.11 and 1.12 where the candidate's attitude to the family is explored. The problem ends with the candidate's own attitudes being tested.

Case 2

Answers

Mrs Richardson is a 32-year-old lady who married for the second time two years ago. She was delivered of a healthy baby boy, James, five months previously after a normal pregnancy. She has two girls, aged seven and five, from her previous marriage, but they now live with their father.

She telephones you at 10.00 pm one night, telling you that James has been passing bright blood in his stools for the past 24 hours, though does not appear to have been distressed.

2.1 Outline your management, giving reasons for your actions.

Visit required: essential to visit any child of this age as he
    may be seriously ill yet show few symptoms.
Possible diagnoses:
    gastroenteritis
    intussusception
    rectal prolapse
    non-accidental injury
    rectal polyp
    proctitis   4
Obtain history
    Physical
        Nature of bleeding: quantity/nature/site (on or in stool, or
            just in nappy)
        Feeding: breast/bottle/solids
            recent habits:? off food, ? hungry
        General: ? vomit, ? bowels, diarrhoea or constipation
            (nature of stools)
            general state of child ? irritable, ? colic, ? pain with
                bowel movement
        Past history of child (and her other children)
        Family illness e.g. gastroenteritis.

Social
 Why has mother not got custody of the two older
  children?
 Circumstances of divorce (? non-accidental injury)
 Why call at 10.00 pm for serious problem of 24 hours
  duration?   6
Examine child
 General: well/unwell; temperature; hydration
 Specific: ear, nose and throat
     abdomen (mass, signe de danse)
     anus (tear, proctoscopy with auroscope, rectal
      (little finger) for rectal polyp/mass, blood on
      finger)
Treatment: dependent on findings, options, are:
 if child not well, or has colic, or dehydrated, or other
  significant problem, admit (advise mother on procedure
  and suggest she goes too)
 most self-limiting and require reassurance with
  explanation.
 Ask her to ring again if bleeding persists or worsens.
 Either revisit in morning, or ask her to 'phone.   6
                 —
                 16
     ————————————

James seems well and you can find nothing abnormal on physical
examination and so you decide to do nothing except see James in the
morning. There is no further bleeding and so you take no further
action. You personally see nothing more of James until he is aged 15
months, when his mother brings him to the surgery complaining
that he will not sleep.

2.2 List the main reasons that might explain this behaviour.

Unrealistic parental expectations
Attention seeking behaviour
Constitutional (temperament)
Parental mismanagement (e.g. poor routine, excessive
 visiting of child if he cries)
Parental emotional problems (child scapegoat) e.g. C_2H_5OH,
 marital dysharmony
Hyperactive child
Social/environmental factors e.g. excess noise, sleeping with
 parents/other siblings
Excessive daytime sleeping

Systemic illness (e.g. pain, fever, cough, ?asthma, eczema)
Miscellaneous: inadequate exercise, hunger, night terrors
  (though a bit young).   6

2.3 What options are open to you in his management?

Full history including:
  feeding habits
  bedtime routines and rituals
  developmental progress
  general emotional difficulties
  physical symptoms.
Examination, e.g. temperature, ENT, RS.
Treatment, dependent on cause
  treat systemic illness if present (unlikely)
  counsel mother *re* sleep expectations, child management,
    environment
  enlist help of health visitor
  family/marital therapy if required
  role of sedatives doubtful: might be acceptable to give short
    course to re-establish sleep pattern. NB may make child
    hyperexcitable.   6
                                                                      ___
                                                                       12

Mrs Richardson brings James back to see you in three weeks saying
that he is still sleeping badly. She tells you that a friend of hers had
sent her some sleeping medicine which she had given James with
good effect, allowing the family the first quiet night for weeks. She
asks you to prescribe some for James.

2.4 How might you respond to this request?

1 Prescribe as requested
2 Prescribe alternative medicine of your choice
3 Refuse request
4 Counsel on sleep management (and variations)
5 Demonstrate empathy/sympathy
6 Explain disadvantages of medication:
      transience of effect
      habituation
      daytime drowsiness
      hyperexcitability
      other side effects.   5

2.5 What action would you take and why?

Option 1 not acceptable
Option 2 acceptable for short term (e.g. 1 week) if
    combined with 4
Option 6 important
Option 3 acceptable if combined with 4
Option 5 should appear
Options 4+5 most acceptable.

Mrs Richardson seems reluctant to take your advice. You do not see
her in the surgery for a year. This time she tells you that James
always has a runny nose, is snuffly, and tends to snore when he
does sleep.

2.6 List the main causes for these symptoms.

Causes
    Allergy
    Catarrhal child (chronic overproduction of mucus)
    Enlarged adenoids
    Nasal blockage (foreign body), especially if unilateral
    Recurrent upper respiratory tract infections
    Normal child with overanxious mother
    Rhinitis medicamentosa
    Septal deviation.

2.7 Outline your management.

Management
History
    past history of ac OM etc.
    onset, duration, relief
    family history of allergy
    possible allergens, e.g. house dust mite, feathers
    hearing test by health visitor.
Mother's understanding, expectations and beliefs
Examination of
    ears for fluid
    nasal airways and septum
    tonsils
    glands
    respiratory system

hearing
adenoids?
? further investigation, e.g. X-ray postnasal space and
    allergy testing: probably not much use   4

Treatment
    education
    self limiting
    not antibiotics unless acute otitis media
    remove foreign body if present
    symptomatic relief
    nasal decongestant not recommended
    systemic antihistamines (might help sleep disturbance!)
    consultant referral—? adenoidectomy especially if deaf.   4
                                                        11

Mrs Richardson replies that she has another (different) friend whose
child had similar symptoms which were cured by tonsillectomy. She
asks you to refer James for tonsillectomy.

2.8 What main points would you like to discuss with her?

Concept of catarrhal child
Expectations of mother
Reasons for tonsillectomy in general
Risks and problems of tonsillectomy
Natural regression of symptoms as child grows
Effect of operation/separation/hospital admission on child's
    psyche
Discussion of friend's problems probably fruitless
Merit/demerits of second opinion
Doubts of your management
Repeated minor illness in child may be presenter of family
    tensions/splits: enquiry along these lines may be fruitful,
    in view of past presenting symptoms.   7

You are on call one Saturday a few weeks later when Mrs
Richardson rings you at home. Apparently her two daughters were
supposed to have spent their usual weekend with her but have
failed to arrive. She is particularly worried as her ex-husband has

seemed under some strain recently and she had noticed some bruises on one of the girls at their last visit.

2.9 What options are open to you in managing this situation?

1   Contact husband directly.
2   Wait till next weekend (or next week) and assess then
3   You or her contact
      social services
      police
      NSPCC
      health visitor
4   Visit husband yourself (but only if he is patient of practice)
5   Do nothing—risk of missing non-accidental injury or other familial injury
6   Provide counselling for Mrs Richardson
7   Suggest she contacts solicitor now or next week
8   Contact Family Law Association or equivalent.   6

2.10 Which would you favour and why?

Options variable, but should be aware that non-accidental injury may be happening and shouldn't miss opportunity to help with this. Options 7 and 8 probably best as husband is probably contravening access orders from courts.

_____

The family move away shortly after, but move back into your area when James is aged 11 and re-register on your list. Mrs Richardson rings asking for a visit for James. He has a painful right knee and is not very well. You find that he has a temperature of 38 deg., his right knee is painful on active and passive movement and there seems to be a mild effusion. There are no other joint signs.

2.11 What are the main differential diagnoses?

Septic arthritis/osteomyelitis
Trauma with coincidental systemic symptoms
Transient arthritis (irritable joint)
Acute juvenile arthritis (Still's disease)
Rheumatic fever
Haemarthrosis
Systemic illness, e.g. rubella, tuberculosis, other viruses.   4

2.12 What options are open to you in his management?

1 Observe at home
2 Consult with paediatrician on 'phone
3 Domiciliary visit
4 Admit directly
5 Further tests at home
      e.g. FBC, ESR, Rheumatoid tests
      X-ray
      aspirate?   5

2.13 Which would you favour and why?

Options must take into account risk of leaving septic arthritis
   without adequate treatment, therefore some consultation
   with paediatrician mandatory, either via 1, 2 or 3. $\frac{4}{13}$

After discussion of the problem with the local paediatrician, James is
admitted to the local hospital. This is his first hospital admission,
and he is clearly very nervous about it. The next day you are rung by
a member of the local branch of the National Association for the
Welfare of Children in Hospital. She tells you that she was concerned at the distress James showed on admission and asks to
attend a team meeting in your Health Centre to discuss ways in
which children might be prepared for admission to hospital.

2.14 What areas might be covered at this meeting?

Points which need to be got over to patient*
   Factual explanations of reasons for admission and what will
         happen
      ward routines, privacy, toileting, etc.
      other children
      investigations: what and why
   Fears mainly of pain, procedures and mutilation
   The better informed the lower the incidence of emotional
         disturbance
   Allow question asking
   Appreciation of need to be child as well as verging on adult
         at his age

Estimate length of admission
Give some idea of probable outcome of illness.   7
General guidance
  Parental
    facilities available
    importance of staying with child and regular visiting
  Political pressures
  Join National Association for the Welfare of Children in
      Hospital
  School visits to hospitals
  Playworkers in hospitals   6
                                                                   ___
                                                                    13

James is discharged from hospital with a diagnosis of juvenile
chronic rheumatoid arthritis (ankylosing spondylitis type).

**2.15 What points would you want to discuss with the
Richardsons at your next meeting with them?**

What had they been told in hospital
Understanding and expectations and fears of illness
James' understanding, expectations and fears
Treatment regime
Drugs: nature, why, compliance, side effects
Exercise
Physiotherapy
Prognosis
Genetic implications
How it will affect whole family
Careful follow-up by GP
Easy access to GP over problem, e.g. when to consult etc.
Schooling, employment and future problems
Aids if required
Build up personal relationship
General problems of chronic illness in children
Brush up own knowledge!   10

Commentary

The MEQ about the Richardsons begins with a late visit but it is a complex situation which is reflected in the mark of 16%. Mrs Richardson is married for the second time but does not have custody of her children from the first marriage: this has to be taken into account when devising a management strategy. In questions 2.4 and 2.5, 9% is given when the candidate's response to a patient request is tested: the candidate's attitude is being explored.

When the question of non-accidental injury is raised in questions 2.9 and 2.10 the candidate's decision making is tested: to score well he has to consider the options and implications in bringing in other agencies. In the following section about the management of the painful knee the discussion of the options with a decision being made scores 9% with the differential diagnosis 4%. The problem ends with the development of a management plan for James's long term care.

Case 3

Answers

Mr C aged 52, and Mrs C, aged 48 years, have been patients in the practice for many years. They live in a council house, and have 3 married daughters nearby. Without warning, Mr C suffers a cere-brovascular accident with L hemiplegia. He is lucid, articulate, and continent. You visit him within an hour of the onset.

3.1 What factors would determine your plan of management?

General fitness:
    blood pressure, blood chemistry, respiratory and cardiac
      state, weight.   3
Mental outlook:
    optimistic, determined to get well.   2
Domestic situation:
    possibility of house care (fitness and willingness of wife);
      suitable accommodation.   6
Home care resources:
    physiotherapy, nursing, aids. $\frac{3}{14}$

3.2 What would you tell Mr and Mrs C regarding prognosis?

Honest appraisal of situation, awaiting outcome of natural
    recovery and physiotherapy. Underline plus points,
    such as lucidity, speech, continence.   5

After several weeks of physiotherapy, Mr C's hemiparesis remains complete, and he has developed severe pain in the left leg at night.

3.3 What causes of the pain would you consider?

He has what appear to have been 2 grand mal seizures at night,
    and Mrs C is unable to sleep.
Contracture of flexor muscles.   2
Sciatic pain derived from posture.   2
Circulatory restriction, causing cramp.   2
Arthritis. $\frac{2}{8}$

3.4 What are your options in dealing with this situation?

Arrange brain scan as area of cerebral damage may be
　　extending.

Consider use of anti-epileptic therapy. Discuss with
　　consultant physician.　　　　　　　　　　　　　　　4

Consider relief for Mrs C at night by night nurse, daughter,
　　close friend.　　　　　　　　　　　　　　　　　　3

Possible admission to hospital for Mr C for stabilization.　　2
　　　　　　　　　　　　　　　　　　　　　　　　　　9

Mr C settles down, and attends a Day Centre twice a week. He is
very demanding and Mrs C shows signs of strain. She tells you she
has bouts of perspiration, and frequency of bowel and bladder.
There is apparent weight loss.

3.5 What causes of her condition would you consider at this time?

1	Anxiety state.	3
2	Thyrotoxicosis.	2
3	Infection.	2
4	Malignant disease.	3
		10

3.6 How would you confirm or refute them?

1　Likely to be present, whether or not the cause.　　　　3
2　Check T3, T4, TSH.　　　　　　　　　　　　　　2
3　Temperature, raised pulse, full blood and white count and
　　ESR, possible foci (chest, urinary system).　　　　　3
4　Systematic check of all areas.　　　　　　　　　　3
　　　　　　　　　　　　　　　　　　　　　　　　11

You have several investigations pending for Mrs C, when you are
called at night because she has severe abdominal pain. This has
gone when you arrive, and on examination you find only slight
tenderness in the R flank.

3.7 Do you consider she warrants further investigation at this stage? If so, what?

Suspect relationship with weight loss, etc. Careful check of
　　abdomen with barium enema, barium meal, fibroscopy.　　10

Mrs C's daughter says she thinks her mother is trying to involve her in the care of her father. She has 3 young children and cannot give any more time.

3.8 What is your response to her?

Mrs C needs all the support she can get. Daughter has been great help, could her other sisters give some time, possibly on a rota system. Possible extension of Primary Care support. Take opportunity to discuss mother's health in light of recent symptoms.   10

Mrs C has a further attack next day, and you find her with signs of intestinal obstruction. She is admitted to hospital, where she is found to have carcinoma of ascending colon with spread into liver. She is sent home to her daughter, who is already caring for Mr C. Both parents think Mrs C is cured.

3.9 What is your reaction to Mrs C's discharge from hospital with an optimistic outlook?

Perhaps better if Mrs C had been left with idea that cancer had been removed (she is likely to have feared this diagnosis) but that scarring and adhesions in abdomen might need treatment later. Mr C's comprehension is clear, and it would probably be better if he were told the truth, since he is likely to outlive his wife.   10

3.10 What options do you now have, and which do you favour?

1	Leave well alone.	1
2	Tell Mr C—but how will he converse with Mrs C when she worsens?	2
3	Tell Mrs C—but indicate good operation, with possible upsets during healing.	3
4	Tell both the full story, but consider the effects on two helpless people.	2
	Option 3 appears good compromise	8

Mrs C dies quietly in bed overnight. You find Mr C withdrawn and uncooperative. He will only speak to his young grandchildren.

3.11 What do you think is behind Mr C's behaviour? Indicate its likely progress.

Mr C is now bereft of his wife, on whom he had become dependent. He is likely to go through the usual bereavement process, with additional emotional reactions due to his own disability; anger at Medicine in general for failure to save his wife; his situation away from his own home and familiar things. He may even contemplate suicide. It is probable that, given time, he will regain his former outgoing attitude.   5

Commentary

The MEQ deals with a common problem of deteriorating health in an elderly couple and how the family doctor's management not only involves the old couple but also the other members of the family. In the first questions the domestic situation and the home care resources gain the highest proportion of the marks indicating their importance in general practice. In questions 3.3 and 3.4 the help for Mrs C was as important as the tests being arranged.

Subsequently the test for Mrs C's abdominal pain was considered to be of the same importance as the candidate's response to the daughter's cry for help. After discharge from hospital 18% is awarded for the patient and family management and this deals mainly with the candidate's attitudes to the patient and his family.

Case 4

Answers

Mr and Mrs S lost their only child (aged 17 years) as a result of Hodgkin's Disease. They are now in their mid-sixties. Mr S has recurrent duodenal ulcer symptoms, but refuses investigation. Mrs S has taken sleeping pills since her daughter's death.

4.1 What management choices are available to you dealing with his recurrent acute dyspepsia? Which do you favour, and why?

General	
Discussion of way of life, reduction of stress.	1
Regular meals, 'sensible' diet.	1
Stop smoking.	1
Avoid excess alcohol consumption.	1
Regular hours.	1
Medication	
Alkalies, e.g. aluminium hydroxide.	1
Motility drugs, e.g. metoclopromide.	1
H_2 antagonists, e.g. cimetidine.	1
Specialized	
He has already refused investigation, although it would be helpful to have fibroscopy/barium meal.	2
	10

4.2 What are your views on Mrs S and her night sedation? What advantages/disadvantages do you see in broaching the subject with her?

It is now some years since Mrs S went on sleeping pills. Removal might cause more upset than benefit, assuming drug is mild. Your previous association with their late daughter may have made you a valued friend. Gentle hints may be most successful approach, if she shows no harmful signs of long-term drug consumption.   5

Mr S consults you because of indigestion and tells you his wife is drinking (whisky) heavily, often together with her Nitrazepam. He thinks you should 'do something' about this.

4.3 What choices of reply would you consider?

It is a domestic issue, of no concern to you.	1
Express concern, and seek further details as to amount and frequency and explore why he is worried about it.	2
Suggest that he has a discussion with his wife, indicating his anxiety and encouraging her to see doctor.	2
Go to Mr S's house, and raise the problem with one or both parties.	$\frac{1}{6}$

4.4 Which would you favour, and why?

Suggest that he has a discussion with his wife, indicating his anxiety and encouraging her to see doctor. Would be more likely to lead to a co-operative and constructive approach, as long as consultation was conducted in an open, non-critical manner.	2

Mrs S calls, saying her husband had told her you wanted to see her about her drinking habits.

4.5 What responses are available to you and which do you consider most appropriate?

1	Indicate that Mr S had mentioned his anxiety to you but that you particularly wanted any consultation to be on a voluntary basis.	2
2	Say that consultation would only be worthwhile if she seriously wished to stop drinking.	1
3	Invite her to sit down and tell you why she feels the need to drink alcohol and if she thinks her consumption is excessive.	2
4	Agree that a stiff drink at night is an excellent relaxant.	1
	A combination of 1 and 3 would seem a reasonable approach.	$\frac{2}{8}$

Mr S develops L. homonymous hemianopia, and asks if this event will affect his driving licence. He admits to having two short instances of loss of consciousness in the past month.

4.6 What is your reply?

Indicate the requirements of driving licence as regards vision i.e. to read a licence plate number at 25 yards. Amplify by demonstrating the inherent dangers in driving with reduced peripheral vision. Suggest that he might actually be worse off running a car than using other transport when necessary. 8

4.7 What other limitations do you see in his information?

He has established cerebrovascular disability, and describes two other events of possibly the same aetiology. He may have a source of emboli in the carotid system, or in the heart. 10

4.8 What action, if any, do you consider you should take?

Advise general medical examination, checking for hyper-tension, arrhythmias, valvular defects, carotid bruits. Also full-blood examination—? polycythaemia; CNS deficits. In view of his previous objection to investigation, it may not be possible to proceed to scans and arteriograms.   8
                                                                    ⎯⎯
                                                                    26

A year later Mr S has a cerebrovascular accident with sensory aphasia but no loss of motor function. He is unable to understand when spoken to, and gives unintelligible replies.

4.9 What courses of action are open to you, and which would you favour?

Admit to hospital, for assessment.   2
Observe at home, possibly with a domiciliary consultation by specialist.   4
Use drugs claimed to improve cerebral circulation such as Naftidrofuryl oxalate (Praxilene). Aspirin contraindicated with duodenal ulcer history.   2
Observe at home, possibly with a domiciliary consultation by specialist would appear to be reasonable, depending on how well Mrs S could cope.   2
                                                                    ⎯⎯
                                                                    10

Three weeks later, Mrs S phones at 7.00 am to tell you her husband has been vomiting all night and is apparently in pain.

4.10 On your way to the patient, what possibilities would occur to you as to the cause of this event?

Recurrence of acute duodenal ulcer type symptoms.	2
Extension of cerebro-vascular disorder.	2
Other unrelated causes, e.g. obstruction, glaucoma, renal stone, gall stone.	2
	$\overline{6}$

On arrival at Mr S's house, you find the patient collapsed and evidence of considerable haematemesis. You have him admitted to hospital where he is found to have a perforated duodenal ulcer. He seems to make progress after repair, but suddenly dies on 2nd post-operative day. The hospital asks you to inform his wife and seek permission for a post mortem examination.

4.11 What is your reaction to this request?

Seems a reasonable manner for hospital to act. Mrs S will receive the news, sudden as it is, better from you. Request for post mortem probably acceptable also, since it appears to have been an unexpected death. It would also be helpful to ascertain the circumstances as far as possible, and hopefully to reassure wife that death was swift and not painful.   8

4.12 What options do you have for dealing with it, which do you choose and why?

1	Tell hospital to contact Mrs S direct.	1
2	Accept message and telephone Mrs S.	1
3	Visit Mrs S and discuss situation.	3
4	Visit Mrs S and discuss situation and contact friend/relative to come to her support.	4
	Option 4. Visit Mrs S and discuss situation and contact friend/relative to come to her support would likely achieve the desired result and maintain security for Mrs S.	$\underline{9}$

4.13 How do you see your role with regard to Mrs S in the near future? Specify her likely problems and your approach to them?

Mrs S will undergo the usual pangs of bereavement. In addition, she now finds herself alone, her daughter and husband dead. She may feel guilty over delaying call to doctor on night of perforation. Doctor's role is to praise her efforts; point out that she maintained her husband in difficult circumstances at home for three weeks, and that his final death resulted from an old ailment which he had refused to have investigated over many years. Maintain contact over a lengthy period, and encourage return to social activities.   10

Commentary

The problem deals with a couple who have previously lost their only child. Mr S has a duodenal ulcer, a condition which has a psychological overlay and this added to his previous loss gives him a fear of hospitals: he refuses investigation. When the husband informs the doctor about his wife's excess drinking six marks are awarded for varying replies to the husband.

After his cerebral incident, Mr S asks about continuing to drive: the handling of this situation with possible actions are of paramount importance and are given 26%. The management following Mr S's death is also extremely important: the dealings with the hospital doctor and the widow being given 27%. This emphasizes the importance of completing all questions as the candidate who does not finish in the time available could only score a maximum of 73% with a mark of 50% therefore doubtful.

Case 5
Answers

Your first patient in Monday morning surgery states that she overheard a stranger discussing her daughter's miscarriage with the
husband of one of your receptionists.

5.1 What do you say to the patient?

This will depend to some extent on whether the patient is extremely angry or mildly annoyed.	1
'I'm sorry to hear that, but I don't think we should jump to the conclusion that it was from our receptionist that the news originated. You know this is a small town, and everyone knows everyone else, and any news tends to circulate fast!'	2
'It would be most out of character for that particular receptionist to be anything other than extremely discrete, but I think I'll have a word with her just to be sure, and to put both our minds at rest. Leave it with me.'	2

5.2 What do you do?

You may have already formed an opinion based on previous knowledge of the receptionist's character and any previous indiscretions.	3
The best thing to do would be to see the receptionist on her own and tell her what the patient said, to establish whether or not confidence has been broken.	3
	11

On confrontation your receptionist states that the subject of the
discussion, namely the girl who miscarried, had been stealing the
thoughts of your receptionist.

5.3 What further aspects of the history would you feel you had to explore bearing in mind you are her doctor as well as her employer.

Worrying as her doctor
That she may be suffering from a psychotic or depressive
    illness and be in need of psychiatric help/medical
    support.   1
Explore
    mood/thought content/delusions/ideas of reference
    sleep pattern
    concentration.
Look for any Schneider's 1st rank schizophrenic symptoms.
Thought insertion/withdrawal
Thought broadcasting
Feelings of passivity
Voices—running commentary.   3
Also enquire about home situation, marital relationship,
    financial problems.   1
That she may be suffering from an organic illness
    e.g. pre-senile dementia
        alcoholic encephalopathy/psychosis
        brain tumour.   2
Would wish to perform general physical as well as full neuro-
    logical examination (including assessment of cognitive
    function).   1
Worrying as her employer
That her symptoms may prevent her from coping with the
    often delicate and always confidential nature of her job, after
    all, a doctor is responsible for his employee's indiscretions. 3
If she has a chronic illness then she may be unable to carry on
    in this job.   1
Explore how the employee feels about this, perhaps suggest-
    ing that she has some time off work.   1
Bear in mind that her delusion(s) are very real to her and she
    may not be susceptible to appeal to reason.   1
                                           14

A consultant opinion states 'I believe your receptionist has schizophrenia'.
   **5.4 What are your obligations in relation to employment in
      this case?**

It would depend on whether there was a clause in her contract
    referring to specific reasons e.g. certain illnesses whereby
    she could be asked to leave/given retirement on medical
    grounds.   2

Certainly as her doctor you would recommend a period off
    work in order to get her symptoms under control, during
    which time as her employer you would pay her Statutory
    Sick Pay.   3
She may be able to carry on with her work when well but if
    symptoms prove difficult to control, you would discuss the
    possibility of her leaving.   1

5.5 What is the drug therapy likely to be in this case?

Either oral or depot phenothiazines.   1
Depot preparations generally preferred as patients delusions
    often prevent them from taking their medication. This can
    be a problem especially when they feel quite well.
Oral phenothiazines frequently used are
    Chlorpromazine (up to 1 G daily in divided doses)
    Thioridazine (up to 200 mg daily in divided doses)   3
        Less sedating than chlorpromazine.
        Less extra pyramidal symptoms.
    Haloperidol tablets (normally 5 mg t.d.s.)
Depot phenothiazines
    Flupenthixol Decanoate (Depixol)
    12.5–40 mg every 2–4 weeks.
    Fluphenazine Decanoate (Modecate)
    12.5–100 mg every 2–6 weeks.
    Haloperidol Decanoate (Haldol Decanoate)   3
    Up to 100 mg every 4 weeks (mild)
        200 mg every 4 weeks (moderate)
        300 mg every 4 weeks (severe)
                              13

Four weeks later your receptionist 'phones you at home when you
are not on duty to tell you she thinks her husband has had a stroke
and could you come right away?

5.6 What do you do?

Assess whether she was in a fit state of mind to cope with
    phoning another doctor (probably not).   1
Ask her how her husband was, asking her to lie him on his side
    and loosen his clothing and ensure he could do himself no
    harm.   1

Then offer to telephone the doctor on call for her, assuring her
that someone would be with her quickly, if your colleague
was busy then you would come yourself. In any case you
would offer to come to see them the next day.   2
Then ring your colleague, putting him in the picture about the
receptionist's psychiatric illness. If you found he was out
then go to the call yourself.   1
All this would depend on whether the practice had a policy
regarding whether or not to attend calls if the patient by-
passes the practice and contacts you directly at home.   1
Irrespective of policies however, one might make the odd
exception for a patient whom you know very well and particularly where the supporting relative (as here) is suffering
from a psychiatric illness.   5
                                                               ——
                                                               11

Having examined your patient (William) you find he is aphasic and
has a dense right-sided hemiparesis and a homonymous hemianopia. His wife pleads with you to admit him to the district general
hospital.

5.7 Write your admission letter below.

Dear Dr Houseman,
Thank you for accepting this previouly fit 55-year-old man
who is the husband of one of our receptionists. He appears   2
to have had a dense (R) hemiparesis with asphasia, of   1
sudden onset this evening. I feel that his wife would be quite
unable to cope with him at home at present, even with full
back-up. She suffers from a mild psychotic illness, and   2
although she is well controlled at present, tends to be easily
upset and copes badly.   4
He is on no present medication and to my knowledge has not
been seen at the Infirmary before.   1
                                                             ——
                                                             10

Signed
Legibly (must contain Name, Address, Telephone no.)

Whilst in hospital William remains doubly incontinent and
dysphasic. His wife tells you that he is being discharged in three
days and wonders what her problems are likely to be.

5.8 What problems do you forsee for both?

She will find him an excessive burden, with his problems
which would be difficult to cope with for the most stable
and coping person. 1

Her own psychiatric problems could well flare up in the face of
such adversity. 3

They will both need a lot of support from
Doctor 1
District Nurse 1
Speech Therapist 1
Social Services 1

A visit to a Day Centre would be a good idea, on a regular basis for
relief. 2

Practically speaking, the District Nurse will give advice on
incontinence aids.

From doctor's point of view, unless visited extremely frequently,
a great increase in requests for visits. 2

The wife will have to be carefully observed and given time to air
her feelings. Her medication may have to be adjusted if
she appears to be relapsing. 2
___
14

William's improvement is very slow.

**5.9 What are the long term stresses likely to be in this house-
hold.**

For William
Frustration with his own predicament, particularly his in-
ability to communicate satisfactorily. 1
May develop depression which may well go unnoticed. 3
Incontinence causes many problems, including embarrass-
ment, social isolation. 1

For Wife
Frustration with husband's inability to commmunicate with her.
Loneliness (he cannot be very good company for her). 1
Depression at her predicament and the fact that she no longer
has the stimulus and company of work. 1
Feeling that she needs more support to deal with physical
problems e.g. incontinence. 1
No more sex life. 1
Not even some signs of improvement in William to give her
hope. 1
Psychotic symptoms may relapse. 1
___
11

After six months there is another flare up of Marjorie's schizophrenia.

5.10 What are the possible causes for this?

Stresses in the home.   1
Failure of Doctor to pay sufficient attention to her as husband's
    problems are so tangible and time consuming.   2
Wife so busy that she has been forgetting to take her pills (if not
    on a depot injection).   2

5.11 What can you do?

Maintain her at home if not too florid.
Adjust medication and consider depot preparation.   3
Increase District Nursing help for husband *or* perhaps arrange
    admission of husband to cottage hospital (if available).
Ask consultant psychiatrist for opinion
  ? admit to psychiatric hospital   2
  ? domiciliary visit
If so, will *either* need to admit William to hospital too *or* if
    relatives nearby willing to move in and look after him,
    may be better for him to remain in his normal
    environment. $\frac{1}{11}$

You are managing both patients at home.

5.12 What other forms of support can you make use of in this situation?

District Nurses (for William)   1
Social Services and any appropriate aids available   1
Health Visitor   1
Community Psychiatric Nurse (for M)   1
Voluntary Visitors if they don't have many visitors
M especially could be suffering mostly from loneliness $\frac{1}{5}$

Commentary

At the beginning of the problem about confidentiality the answer to
the patient who makes the complaint is more extensive than the

decision about what action to take, but the latter is considered more important and therefore awarded more marks. Question 5.3 looks at the problem from both the doctor's and employer's point of view and high marks are awarded as this is the focal point of the problem.

Note that only 7% is given in question 5.5 for an extensive drug regime: this confirms the lower priority given to knowledge in the MEQ. In question 5.6 watch the trap of giving one answer, e.g. 'Yes, I'll come right away'. The various options are sought with what the doctor would actually do having considered these options.

The importance of communication is shown with the relatively high mark given to the admission letter. The problem ends by showing how the family doctor is involved in caring for both husband and wife and the problems this can lead to. Appropriate use of the practice team scores good marks.

Case 6

Answers

Elizabeth Vernon is 76 years old and lives in a modern council bungalow with her 79-year-old husband. Twelve years ago she had a lobectomy for bronchiectasis. On a home visit at her request she tells you she has been more short of breath recently.

6.1 What other aspects of the history would you wish to elucidate?

Has she had a cough *or* increased sputum *or* change in colour of sputum?	1
As she is more short of breath, is she short of breath at rest, or how far can she walk before becoming short of breath?	1
Is this symptom due to infection, is she/has she been pyrexial ill in bed off food.	1
For how long has she noticed this deterioration: days/weeks/months?	1
Has she lost weight?	1
Is she/has she been a smoker?	1
Is her breathlessness a problem through the night? How many pillows does she sleep with at night?	1
Have her ankles been swollen?	1
? Haemoptysis	1
Have there been any stresses at home to cause her worry?	1
Does her chest feel tight/wheezy when she is in bed?	1
Has she had any chest pains?	1
	$\overline{12}$

On examination she has widespread wheezing with a prolonged expiratory phase.

6.2 What are the four most likely diagnoses. List in order of preference.

1	Chronic obstructive airways disease.	3
2	Late onset asthma.	3

3	Chest infection.	1
4	Cardiac failure.	1
		8

Mrs Vernon seems somewhat upset and depressed during your consultation.

6.3 What might be the possible environmental causes for this?

Marital discord, recent or longstanding.	2
Her husband may need a lot of care and she is exhausted.	2
May be unhappy in her house as it is a modern council bungalow. Have they moved there recently away from old friends?	2
Because of her respiratory problem, is she less able to get to see friends/go to the shops/are the shops very far away?	2
Has she seen much of her family recently?	2
	10

It transpires her additional worry is her husband who has been wandering at night around the house and she isn't sleeping as a result of this.

6.4 What is your management plan?

See husband and examine him thoroughly	
to assess whether he has a confusional state/dementia and	
whether there is a correctable cause e.g.	
drug induced	
infective	
hypothyroid	
Parkinsonism	3
to take this a step further may admit him to Cottage Hospital	
to observe his behaviour *and* to give Mrs V a rest	3
attempt to treat cause of husband's wandering to alleviate	
her worry.	3
? sedate husband nocté, but this could cause problems of its	
own.	3
	12

A detailed examination reveals him to be a moderately demented old man who appears well-nourished, not clinically anaemic and nothing abnormal is found in his urine.

6.5 What investigations would it be reasonable to carry out at this stage?

FBC/ESR	1
Urea and electrolytes.	1
Random blood glucose.	1
T4	1
? chest X-ray depend on availability.	1
	$\frac{1}{5}$

The following day Mrs Vernon's daughter telephones you to ask what you propose to do about her mother's situation since she lives five miles away and is therefore unable to help.

6.6 What do you tell her?

Reassure her that you are actively involved in the situation and attempt to solve certain problems.	3
Suggest that although she is not able to help in an emergency at night, she might help by visiting her parents a little more often during this time.	3
Say that you might suggest a home help which would give Mrs V more rest through the day.	2
	$\frac{}{8}$

The situation gradually deteriorates at home over the next six months. The main problem being the worsening dementia of Mr Vernon.

6.7 What options have you for helping the situation?

Attempt to evaluate what is the single greatest problem. Is it Mr V's dementia?	1
If so, ? admit him to hospital temporarily/permanently.	2
If Mrs V needs more help, involve social services to arrange home help.	1
If neither is desperately ill/impaired, ? suggest move to sheltered warden-controlled accommodation.	2
If more impaired, ? move to residential home (both).	2

Crossroads Scheme may be able to arrange someone to come
    and give Mrs V a few hours relief if he needs constant
    attendance.   2

Persuade daughter to help more.   1

? Health Visitor may be able to assist.   1

If Mr V needs nursing care/help with baths, district nurse
    could help.   1
                        13

While in the local geriatric unit it is discovered that Mr Vernon has
maturity onset diabetes mellitus.

**6.8 What problems do you foresee when discharge home is
imminent?**

Mrs Vernon may be worried about problems she may
    encounter
    will she have to inject insulin?
    will certainly have to test urine/supervise diet.
    she may be feeling much better in herself after her rest, and
        worried that all will deteriorate again when he is home.   5

You will have to visit frequently in order to help maintain his
    diabetic control

and may not yet have received a hospital discharge summary
    with details of his regimen.

You may need to ask the district nurse to help with his
    injections if he is on insulin.   3

Mr Vernon may not have a good understanding of his problem
    due to dementia *or* poor communication in hospital and
    be worried about what pills to take, what to eat, who will
    do his injections when at home.   3
                        11

**6.9 What would your management plan be for Mr Vernon
providing he was fit to remain at home?**

Follow up his diabetic control yourself either checking at home
    or in the surgery depending on whether or not he was fit.   2

Involve wife in helping him with urine testing, diet, injections
    if appropriate.   2

In the short term, check random blood glucose weekly, urine
    daily.   2

Regular chiropody.   2

Check blood pressure/urine for protein every 3 months or so
    and go on to check U+E if any abnormality.   1
Check retinae for any evidence of retinopathy and plan regular
    follow-up with pupils dilated.   1
Could contact dietician if wanted advice about diet.   _1_
                                                                         11

Bearing in mind that Mrs Vernon will carry out much of the routine
management,

**6.10 what specific advice would you give Mrs Vernon about
    looking after her diabetic husband?**

Explanation in simple terms of diabetes.   2
The aim is to maintain reasonable control of his blood sugar.   1
It is important to recognize signs that his sugar is getting too
    low: he may feel sweaty, dizzy, palpitations.   1
If this happens be ready to give him milk, sugar lumps or
    dextrose tablets.   1
He may pass out, if so call doctor.
It is not so obvious if the sugar is running too high.
This will show up in the water tests, and takes a longer time to
    develop. Always let doctor know if the urine tests start to
    show sugar.   2
Never allow him to miss a meal as he may go 'hypo'.   1
Make sure you never run too low on insulin, tablets, resting
    tablets/stix, as appropriate.   1
Never be afraid to give doctor a ring to ask for advice.   _1_
                                                                         10

Commentary

The importance of the history is shown early, diagnoses in general
practice can often be made from this alone. This is reflected in 12%
being awarded for this section and only 8% for the four most likely
diagnoses. The relatively heavy weighting given to the environmental causes for her upset reflects its importance in general
practice.

As the case develops the marking scale gives a greater importance
to the daughter's 'phone call than to the investigations for the
father. This reflects the bias towards problem solving, i.e. what is
being tested in the MEQ.

When one looks at the scoring for the management of diabetes (last three sections): out of 32% only about one-third deals with textbook knowledge of diabetes with management of the situation at home getting greater priority. Decision making and problem solving in the candidate are being tested.

Case 7

Answers

Mrs Cassidy had an iron deficiency anaemia fifteen years ago which responded well to therapy. She is now aged 55 and one month ago consulted your partner with tiredness and lassitude. Only one line is recorded in the notes stating that she was given in iron preparation and diazepam. She consults you asking for a repeat prescription.

7.1 How do you handle this situation?

Check old notes to see if any information on anaemia 15 years ago. Suppress irritation over lack of clinical notes, partner had prescribed iron without examining patient or checking blood. Ask how long doctor said she would be on therapy. Assess current situation: is she any better with therapy? Did she have any other complaint or problems when seen one month ago. Take full history and examine. Check FBC, ESR.

Do not criticize partner to patient but say to patient that you need tests to fully assess the situation.

Document all of above fully in notes.   5

7.2 What do you say to your partner?

This depends entirely on your relationship with your partner.
Avoid judgemental statements and suppress irritation.
Ask partner if he remembered seeing her and details of the content of the consultation.
Explain own course of action and ask him if he agrees with this.
Mention tactfully that to-day's consultation would have been easier if he'd written more in the notes.
This may open door to a meaningful discussion of the importance of good clinical notes. $\frac{4}{9}$

You decide to check her blood. You repeat the prescription and arrange to see her in one week. The laboratory phone you in the late afternoon to say that the Hb is 11.9 G% with a film suggestive of chronic granulocytic leukaemia.

7.3 How would you handle this situation?

Ask to speak to consultant haematologist to discuss further course of action. Further action would depend on his response but contact should be made with Mrs Cassidy. You could phone her to tell her that she is anaemic and could she call to see you to-morrow.

You could visit her at home but this may alarm both her and the family.

On the other hand it would show the family how much you care and would allow you to assess the home situation.

Tell her she requires further investigation but at present there is no cause for alarm.   5

Answer questions on the nature of the condition, treatment available, outlook and help possible from primary care team.

Explain what the hospital doctor is likely to do.

Take opportunity to prepare the way for further discussion with the family.

Document all of this in case note.

Discuss diagnosis with partner. $\frac{3}{\frac{8}{}}$

_____

You re-visit Mrs Cassidy to say that you have arranged a hospital admission for the following day. You inform her about this and she asks 'Is there anything to worry about?'

7.4 How do you respond to this?

No—the blood test showed an abnormality which requires further investigation before the seriousness of the situation can be assessed. Stress that the suspected condition is not fatal and that treatment is available. She will be in expert hands and that you will be happy to advise her when required.

Allow patient to ask questions and voice fears.

If asks *re* prognosis admit that you do not know exact figures but you will be prepared to find out and give encouragement about new forms of treatment.   4

She then asks if she can carry on with her work in the College kitchens.

7.5 What advice do you give?

No reason at all to give up work as long as she feels fit to continue. Best to take time off until the investigations are completed. Find out what job entails and offer to speak to supervisor.

Suggest SC_1 initially and reassess her in one week.

Try to keep morale high. If she asks you what she writes on line, suggest 'anaemia—being investigated'.
Reassure her that hospital will issue sick notes if necessary. $\dfrac{4}{8}$

Her hospital admission confirmed the diagnosis of chronic granulocytic leukaemia. Mrs Cassidy was commenced on busulphan 4 mg daily with ferrous sulphate 200 mg TID. She has also to take allopurinol 100 mg TID. You call to see her at home and learn that she has been given no information about her illness in hospital.

7.6 How do you react to this?

Suppress your irritation at the hospital's poor management. Tell her that hospital sometimes doesn't tell the patient since they feel that the GP with his knowledge of the family is better equipped to tell them. Could be helpful to 'phone the hospital and find out exactly what is going on.
Explain
   diagnosis: attempt to explain basics of leukaemia.
   ? prognosis: guarded until one sees how she responds to drug therapy. Mention therapy available with side effects especially reduced resistance to infection.

Explain role of hospital and primary care team.   5

7.7 What would you say to Mr and Mrs Cassidy?

That you are available for any problem. Gauge what you feel, what they want to know at present.
Explore: feelings of anger, grief, anxiety and stress.

Ask how family have reacted. Is employer keeping job open?
  Is she worse off when not working?
If they are genuinely inquisitive then tell them that Mrs
  Cassidy has a form of cancer of the blood which older people
  get but which is treatable with drugs and has a good
  prognosis. Great care has to be taken in the use of the word
  leukaemia as it has a stigma attached to it.
You indicate that you will await hospital report.
Ask what support they get from family, friends, church.   6
                                                            ──
                                                            11
                    ─────────────────

Mrs Cassidy made a satisfactory clinical response and returned to
work. One evening Mr Cassidy and his 30-year-old son come to see
you at the surgery. They ask what the future holds for Mrs Cassidy.
  7.8 What would you say?

Offer sympathy and support. State that this is a relatively
  benign form of cancer which responds to therapy. However
  she will require regular medical supervision for the rest of
  her life. She requires prompt treatment of any infective
  condition.
Find out how things are at present. Are they coping?
If well, dwell on this and help to boost morale. Point out that
  the treatment can lead to a long period of symptom free
  existence.
Involve son in decision making and allow time for Mr Cassidy
  and son to talk.   6

They also ask for guidance on how much she should be allowed to
do.
  7.9 Outline your response.

'Treat her as if she hadn't had a blood test'. She should be
  allowed to continue at work. Over-protection can lead to
  irritation. If barriers are placed in her way then her own
  perception of the disease may change and could lead to
  depression about the situation.
Find out how everyone is coping.   5
                                                            ──
                                                            11
                    ─────────────────

Mrs Cassidy continues to do well carrying out her work and duties at home. She has several urinary tract infections over a four year period and these respond to the appropriate antibiotic.

Mrs Cassidy consults you one evening complaining about acute pain in the middle toe of her (R) foot.

7.10 Discuss the possibilities.

This will depend on history and examination.
Trauma should be obvious.
Vascular, either embolic or peripheral vascular disease.
Neurological: peripheral neuropathy.
Inflammatory: gout as a drug side effect.
Infective
Neoplastic, which is unlikely.
Psychosomatic and therefore an excuse for counselling on
other matters   5

7.11 How would you manage this situation?

After an appropriate history and examination check notes,
hospital letters and current medication.
X-ray, check FBC, ESR, Uric Acid, Platelets and
Immunoglobulin. Discuss how she is managing. Ask *re*
family.
Ask Mrs Cassidy what she thinks is wrong.
Treat with non-steroidal anti-inflammatory drugs until results
available. Consider outpatient appointment.
When results available consider anti-platelet agent.
Explain diagnosis.
Arrange follow-up. $\underline{5}$
                                                                              $\underline{10}$

The foot pain responded to aspirin and persantin therapy. Mrs Cassidy attends you on a regular basis and when aged 62 at a routine appointment she complains of lethargy and tiredness with marked weakness in her legs. She asks you if she should give up her work

7.12 Suggest a differential diagnosis for her symptoms.

? Acute on chronic leukaemia. Could be worsening of
leukaemia with development of anaemia.
Neurological: myasthenia gravis, motor neurone disease.

Endocrine: hypothyroidism or diabetes mellitus.
Psychiatric: depression a possibility.
Psychosomatic: not coping with work and looking for a reason
    to stop.   4

7.13 Discuss a management plan.

Take full history regarding duration of symptoms and
    localization of weakness. Distinguish claudication from
    weakness. Look for symptoms of depression. Ask *re*
    problems at work, attitude to work and current situation at
    home.
Full clinical examination especially peripheral pulses and
    neurological.
Check FBC, ESR, U & E, LFT's. Thyroid function tests.
Refer if appropriate.
Explain to patient what you think and what you are doing.
Arrange follow-up. $\frac{5}{9}$

At her next hospital attendance the marked weakness affecting her
legs is noted. Examination of the central nervous system is negative
and the consultant thinks that she may be depressed. You receive
a note suggesting mianserin 30 mg nocté.
7.14 How do you respond to this?

A difficult situation—who is responsible for the patient?
Did you think she was depressed? On what evidence did the
    haematologist make the diagnosis. Make own assessment of
    situation and if you agree then prescribe. If not then 'phone
    and discuss the matter with the specialist. Should you seek
    the opinion of e.g. a psychiatrist or a neurologist?
Explain to patient what you are doing.
Seek husband's opinion *re* depression.   4

One week later Mr Cassidy calls to see you extremely worried about
his wife. He feels that there is something far wrong.

7.15 What do you say to him?

Express sympathy and concern but allow him to vent his
  feelings. Use open ended questions to find out exactly what
  is worrying him. He may be able to enlighten you about her
  work, her home situation and thus give you a more objective
  view.
Very important to maintain his confidence and to reassure him
  that you are treating the problem with the utmost
  seriousness and urgency.
Make sure that Mr Cassidy is not the patient presenting his
  wife's problems hoping that you will notice his problems.
You may want to suggest to him that there may be cause for
  concern. $\frac{5}{9}$

You decide that she requires neurological investigation and she is
admitted to hospital where the diagnosis of hydrocephalus
secondary to cerebral atrophy is made. When allowed home Mrs
Cassidy can just get about.

7.16 Outline the management problems at this stage.

Physical
Mrs Cassidy:
  dressing, toileting, getting to bed, bathing
  ability to perform household duties
  ability to work.
Is there need for home help, district nurse, social worker,
  occupational therapist, physiotherapist, health visitor?
Finance: ? mobility allowance, ? non-contributing invalidity
  pension, ? attendance allowance.
Emotional: Is she depressed, etc.?
Social: Confined to home: does she read, have TV, any
  hobbies?
Allow time to express feelings of anger, fear etc.
Mr Cassidy:
  Is he able to cope? Can family help?
  Is a nurse required to sit at night?
  Can he take time off work?
Visit regularly and act in supportive role.   4

Mr Cassidy who is aged 61 and is a storeman suggests that he must
retire as his wife requires his full-time care.

7.17 How do you respond to this?

Allow Mr Cassidy to express worries. Explore his feelings of
   anger, grief, guilt and anxiety.
Discuss help from primary care team, meals-on-wheels, home
   help.
Discuss diagnosis and prognosis with him. Try to dissuade
   him from stopping work as prognosis is poor and work
   could be useful in a therapeutic manner.
Offer Med 3 'Nervous strain'.
You could offer to contact firm to explain situation.
Arrange follow-up. $\frac{4}{8}$

There is considerable deterioration in Mrs Cassidy's condition over
the following month: she now has a virtual spastic paraplegia of her
lower limbs. Her husband has insisted on retirement to look after
her.

7.18 What support can Mr and Mrs Cassidy be given?

Continuing care from primary care team
Personal support and regular visiting from GP
Regular nursing care, commode, incontinence pads, etc
? Wheel chair
? night nursing
physiotherapy if needed
occupational therapist
bath aids if needed
Home help, meals-on-wheels.
GP from practice should always be available for patient   4
Finance:
   attendance and mobility allowances if applicable.
   grant for laundry or washing machine.
Ask Social Work Department to advise Mr Cassidy on this.
When visiting allow time to sit and listen.
Enquire whether priest (or equivalent) is attending to their
   spiritual needs.
Involve family to provide support. Also neighbours.
Remember possibility of hospitalization if family are
   distressed and not coping with situation despite all the
   help being provided. A hospice may be more appropriate. $\frac{4}{8}$

Mrs Cassidy dies one week later and her husband is very upset by the death.

7.19 What are the immediate problems for Mr Cassidy?

Coping with the acute grief reaction. Uncertainty of the practical problems of dealing with death, e.g. funeral parlour, burial, who to inform etc.

Stages of bereavement

1   Shock, numbness and can't cope.
2   Anger and blame of himself, family, GP, others.
3   Realization and hopelessness.
4   Gradual acceptance and recovery.

The time scale varies for each but must watch for abnormal reactions. Now is isolated and lonely since he has retired. Poverty as he only has pension. At increased risk of physical and mental illness, also suicide. Could feel guilty about not having looked after wife well enough.   5

7.20 What help can you give him?

Arrange regular follow-up as this man needs support.
Tell him how well he looked after his wife and that she would now want him to lead a normal life.
Allow him to express his feelings of grief, anxiety, guilt and failure.
If he won't attend surgery, visit at home.
Ask district nurse and health visitor who visited Mrs Cassidy to visit Mr Cassidy (they often learn about problems which the doctor doesn't realize).
Contact other members of family to support father. (Hopefully they may already be doing this.)
Try to avoid sedatives and hypnotics (but these may be of use in some patients).
Explain the grief reaction.
Be available and understanding. $\frac{4}{9}$

Commentary

The first three pages test how the doctors deal with the difficult situations, firstly difficulties with his partner and secondly how much bad news should the doctor convey to the patient when a diagnosis is fairly certain but not confirmed and thirdly how he handles searching questions from the patient. This gives a total of 25% and contains little clinical medicine.

After her discharge from hospital, skills handling the patient and her family are dealt with in the next two pages (further 22%). With the development of acute toe pain in the following two pages dealing with the clinical situation is important but only attract 19%.

The remainder deals with the GP coping in difficult circumstances, involving the practice team and supporting the family, especially the husband, after the death of his wife. Overall knowledge of clinical medicine attracted less than one quarter of the total mark. The majority of the marks were for the skills of decision making and communicating with patients and relatives. Management plans when dealing with a difficult area formed the basis of this problem.

Case 8

Answers

Mr James is a 40-year-old electrician who has just joined your practice. He consults you one evening stating that he wishes to lose weight. He is 170 cm and weighs 120 kg.

8.1 What other information do you require?

Reason for change of practice: ? new to area, ? change of job, ? quarrel with previous GP.
Find relevant details about him with new patient proforma. Why does he want to lose weight now? What is his exercise/ eating pattern? Find out *re* health determinants (smoking, alcohol and blood pressure).
Does he have any physical symptoms, e.g. dyspnoea.
Does he have psychological problems, e.g. image problem.
? Pressures from wife or at work.
? Previous attempts at weight loss. ? Recent weight changes.   6

8.2 How do you deal with this problem?

Establish both rapport and that motivation for losing weight is present. Discuss reasons for obesity, i.e. intake is greater than expenditure of energy. Assess dietary habits.
Counsel patient to encourage realistic aims. Explain that you do not use drugs because of
side effects
danger of addiction and
lack of persistent effect.
Advise three meals daily with calorie intake of 1200–1500.
Avoid high calorie foods: substitute alternatives and advise graded increase in exercise.
Increase motivation by seeing dietician, attending self-help group e.g. weight watchers or health visitor.
Enlist family support (see wife at next visit).
Exclude medical causes of obesity.
Explain that weight loss is vital to future health.
Review in 1 month. $\frac{8}{14}$

Mr James lives with his wife in a local authority house. They have no family. You do not see him for two years when he consults you about thirst and polyuria. You test his urine and find 2% glycosuria but no ketones. You note his weight is now 122 kg and he continues to smoke 20 per day.

8.3 Outline your management plan at this stage.

Repeat urinalysis on freshly produced specimen.

Arrange urgent blood biochemistry (urea and electrolytes, blood sugar).

Also chest X-ray.

If no electrolyte imbalance then keep at home off work.

Exclude precipitating causes, e.g. liver disease.

Explain that diabetes is causing his symptoms and that this is directly related to his obesity. If he loses weight then this might be sufficient to control symptoms.

Carry out full examination: cardio-vascular system, respiratory system, central nervous system, fundi, peripheral pulses.

Commence sugar free diet and arrange to see dietician. Patient to monitor progress by checking urine twice daily. Review patient daily for a few days then at increasing intervals. If no improvement after several weeks consider oral hypoglycaemic agent (probably metformin because of obesity). If shows no improvement with this consider referral to hospital outpatients.

? Base line ophthalmological opinion.

Wife to be involved in management as soon as possible.

Encourage Mr James to stop smoking. 11

Mrs James calls to tell you that her husband has been drinking heavily for six months. He is now missing time at work especially at the beginning of the week.

8.4 What is the significance of this information?

Previously withheld by patient as has been given without his consent. Could be a factor in his obesity and may suggest poor compliance for therapy in diabetes. May be alcoholic but does he accept what wife says.

Wife is concerned: financial implications, guilt, genuine concern about patient, fear of physical assault. 4

8.5 What further information would you ask Mrs James?

Full drinking history: how long?, how much?, when?, why?,
    ? underlying marital problems, ? mental illness in husband.
Assess effect of drink on her husband, on her, their marriage.
Why is she giving you this information? Can she help?
How do colleagues at work feel about him?
Does he accept that he has a problem?   3

8.6 How would you deal with the problem?

Advise Mrs James to ask her husband to consult alone or as a
    couple. If he won't do this, counsel Mrs James herself:
    supply her with information about local alcohol treatment/
    support groups e.g. Alanon, Woman's refugees. If he comes
    to see you, ask him about intake, check for stigmata of liver
    disease. Take blood for γ GT, LFT's, transaminases and
    blood alcohol.
Try to assess if Mr James has any problems e.g. financial,
    marriage. Warn him of dangers of alcohol excess.
Refer to Council for Alcoholism, Alcoholics Anonymous.
Arrange follow-up.   4
          ————————————   ——
                                            11

Mr James comes to see you at your request. He denies that there is a
problem and states that he has drastically cut his alcohol intake. He
has just applied for a job as an electrician on the oil rigs and is keen to
get this.

8.7 If successful how would this affect the lifestyle of Mr and Mrs James?

Mr James
Drinking not allowed on rigs. ? Increased intake when he is at
    home. ? Possibility of DT's on return to rigs.
Financial state will improve therefore easier to purchase
    alcohol.
Separation could put less strain on marriage when away but
    increased stress when at home.
Diet may be improved on rigs but little relaxation so could put
    on weight.
Discipline of work would be good.   5

Mrs James

Will be left alone as have no children. Is she a coper—more likely to visit doctor with self-limiting illnesses, increased consultations and increased prescriptions.

Would have more money and expectations would increase.

Could be more concerned about husband when she doesn't see him as has lost her 'role'.

Could alienate friends because of increased wealth.

Both

With extra money may want to move to new house.   5
                                                  ──
                                                  10

Three months later Mr James's diabetes is well controlled on metformin 850 mg BD: he has lost 12 kg in weight and states that he feels better than he has done for years. He calls for a medical examination for the oil rigs and you find a blood pressure of 190/105 both lying and standing.

8.8 What do you say to Mr James?

Congratulate him on losing weight. Blood pressure elevated but commonest reason for this is excitement so there is nothing to worry about at present. Further readings are required. However regret that this information has to be passed on to potential employer. Diabetes at present well controlled. Explain nature of hypertension and excellent results of treatment.

Ask patient if he wants to ask anything.   4

8.9 What is your management plan?

Check blood pressure on at least two further occasions.

If normal recheck in six months.

If elevation confirmed, exclude treatable cause, examine looking specifically for target organ involvement (esp. fundi).

Arrange FBC, ESR, urea and electrolytes, electrocardiogram and chest X-ray.

Also urinalysis.

Reinforce need to lose more weight and to stop smoking.

Mention relationship between diabetes and hypertension, the need for life long therapy.

Because of diabetogenic effects of thiazides, commence a cardioselective β-blocker e.g. Atenolol 50 mg daily. Review 2–3 weeks.

$$\frac{7}{11}$$

His blood pressure settles to 140/85 on Atenolol 100 mg daily and you decide that he can work on the oil rigs. His working pattern is two weeks on the rigs then two weeks at home.

8.10 What are the potential problems for Mr James?

Irregular hours (probably 12 on and 12 off) may bring problems with diet and drug compliance. Enforced alcohol abstinence alternating with opportunity for binge drinking.
Marriage will be further stressed.
May be tired as a side effect of β-blockers thus affecting his ability to work. Possibility of hypoglycaemia.
Markedly increased earnings may be spent in inadvisable way. 6

8.11 From the limited information you have about her how do you think Mrs James would cope with such an arrangement?

May be relieved by his absence: relations at home have been strained because of his drinking.
No children so could be lonely.
May have to turn more to friends and neighbours.
Will tend to consult doctor more with self-limiting illness.
However could establish own new independent lifestyle.

$$\frac{5}{11}$$

You do not see him for eighteen months. He consults you one evening with an itch at his (L) ankle.

8.12 How do you handle this consultation?

Assess reason for consultation. Is itch the real reason or a 'passport' to introduce other complaints. Ask him why he hasn't attended for so long. How compliant has he been about diet and medication. What is his alcohol intake. Advise need for annual check for hypertension and diabetes.

Cause of itch
  ? neurodermatitis, ? eczema, ? varicose vein, ? peripheral
    neuropathy.
Allow him to talk about any worries he has.   6

8.13 What are the potential problems?

Continuing worries about compliance.
Current state of drinking and smoking.
Marital problems.
Employment.
Diabetes and hypertension.
Development of ulcer which can be difficult to heal.   6
                                                            ――
                                                             12

Six months later Mrs James calls to tell you that her husband is again drinking to excess. He pays little attention to his diet, has gained 12 kg in weight.

8.14 What action would you take?

Consider underlying causes for consultation.
Offer to see them individually or as a couple.
Find out more about how he spends his days.
Ask Mrs James what she thinks.
Suggest that she tells him about her visit to the surgery.   5

8.15 When Mr James calls to see you, what do you say to him?

Ask him why he has come. Does he recognize that he has a
  problem. Ask about alcohol intake.
Reinforce the use of a planned management for his conditions.
Does he want help. Potential of further marital, financial,
  occupational problems.
Be blunt indicating that he is damaging his health.
Consider Council on Alcoholism, Alcoholics Anonymous.
Arrange follow-up.   6
                                                            ――
                                                             11

You arrange for Mr James to attend for a further appointment at the local diabetic clinic. He is again noted to be hypertensive (BP 165/100). A diuretic is added to his current regime. Two days later Mr James calls at the surgery insisting that he sees you.

At the consultation he demands to know what the future holds for him.

8.16 How do you handle this confrontation?

Acknowledge anger and accept that it may be useful in uncovering underlying problems/anxieties. Ask him why he is annoyed: what particular aspect of management is worrying him. Stress the importance of keeping to appointment system. Indicate that if he follows management than can have healthy life. 3

8.17 Why may he be taking such an attitude?

Could be upset by hospital visit, more treatment, worried about complications. Could have seen ill diabetics. Doesn't like having his life controlled by doctor. Seriousness of situation may just have become apparent: worried about recent poor compliance. Fear of future, ? side effects of medication.

Anxiety/depression. 3

8.18 What is his long-term outlook?

Would seem poor but can't be more exact without precise parameters. Has several risk factors for developing vascular disease, alcohol and poor compliance only add to these problems.

His greatest risk is of developing a myocardial infarction, now the commonest cause of death in adult diabetics. 3

$$\frac{3}{\overline{9}}$$

Commentary

The first page of the problem on Mr James deals with two vague areas: firstly a new patient joining your list and secondly this patient wants to lose weight. Both can be dismissed quickly but this would reflect poor management: their importance is shown in the marking schedule with this page scoring 14%, the highest for any one page in the problem. His management when he is found to be diabetic, although important and reflecting a high degree of knowledge only merits 11%.

The third part reflects a difficult problem when illness is reported by a third person and the GP must decide how he deals with this information. The latter parts of the question test the effect of social factors on the lifestyle of the James's: the good candidate with extensive experience of general practice should score well here. Note that the management plan for hypertension only scores 7%.

Case 9

Answers

Mr John Williams aged 48 has been your patient for ten years. He consults you because of increasing breathlessness over six months. He attributes his symptoms to stopping smoking at that time.

9.1 What do you say in response to this?

Congratulate him on giving up. Agree that when you stop smoking at first quite common to feel a bit stuffed up and therefore short of breath but six months seems a bit long.

Reinforce the health benefits of giving up smoking. Emphasize that dyspnoea is distressing and that we must find the cause of it.   4

9.2 What further information do you require?

Severity of breathlessness: onset, progress, ? Orthopnoea, ? PND.

Associated cough or spit? Chest pain? Appetite and weight? Fainting? Blood loss? Palpitation? General health? Past medical history? Current drug history? Smoking history? Occupational history?   4

9.3 What examination and tests would you carry out at this initial consultation?

General: ? pallor, central cyanosis, finger clubbing, ankle swelling, cardiovascular system including blood pressure and peripheral pulses.

Respiratory system.

Abdomen.

Investigations
 FBC, ESR
 Chest X-ray
 Electrocardiogram $\frac{6}{14}$

You detect the murmur of aortic stenosis. He is normotensive but grossly overweight (94 kg): this he attributes to stopping smoking.

9.4 What do you say to Mr Williams?

His weight is a bit of a problem: it is common to gain weight after stopping smoking but usually around 7 lb. What weight was he aged 20?

Ask *re* food intake and exercise. Does he eat many sweets or drink excess alcohol? You can hear a heart murmur which is contributing to the breathlessness but it is difficult to assess because of obesity. Has anyone ever mentioned a heart murmur to him?   4

9.5 Outline your management plan.

Advise him to lose weight and offer help if he wants this. Exclude an underlying cause of obesity if required. Educate him about diet and specific types of food. Give diet sheet if required. Refer to other members of practice team if appropriate e.g. dietician or health visitor with special interest.

Give short term target weight.

Refer Cardiologist.

Reinforce cigarette abstention.

Review 10 days.   7
                                                                   ——
                                                                   11

You arrange a cardiological opinion: he is seen by the Registrar who thinks the main problem is severe hypertension (blood pressure 200/120 with normal fundi) and obesity. Electrocardiogram and Chest X-ray negative. Aortic stenosis not haemodynamically significant.

9.6 Comment on the Registrar's opinion.

Unlikely to be correct. Unlikely to have severe hypertension: blood pressure normal when seen in surgery, fundi normal which is very unlikely in severe hypertension. Hypertension should never be diagnosed on one elevated reading.

Patient was referred for specialist opinion which does not seem to have happened.   4

Mr Williams asks you exactly what is wrong with him and can he continue his work as a taxi-driver.

9.7 How do you respond to this?

Reassure him that he can continue work as taxi-driver. (No syncope or angina symptoms); but say there is still some debate

Draw diagram showing him where the block is and why the back pressure causes some pooling of fluid in the lung (and thus dyspnoea).

Although the hospital doctor felt that he had high blood pressure you think this will settle. The most important immediate problem is to lose weight and reduce cardiac load.

Also reassure him that if his blood pressure remains elevated there are now many satisfactory forms of management.

No pills are necessary at present. $\frac{6}{10}$

_____

Mr Williams's blood pressure settles without treatment and he loses 10 kg in weight. The cardiologist discharges him but asks you to re-refer him if there is any deterioration in his symptoms.

The day before one of his routine visits you receive a letter from his sister telling you that he is again smoking 20 per day.

9.8 How do you handle this situation at his next consultation?

Tell him about satisfactory letter from hospital. Then ask:
   How are things?
   Any problems?
   Diet?
   Still off cigarettes?

He will probably admit to restarting but will give you a lower daily number. Reinforce the absolute necessity for no smoking. On no account mention letter from sister.
Reassure him that dyspnoea was unconnected to stopping smoking.   4

9.9 From your experience, discuss the value of health education *re* smoking during the consultation. How might you educate about smoking?

Of some value in the limited time available. A number of patients reduce their smoking as a result of advice but even the most enthusiastic only have a success rate of 5% after one year. More likely to be successful if there is a marked change in their health caused by smoking or someone close has died of a smoking related disease.

Education about smoking consists of posters in the waiting room, straight discussion at consultation with the back up of education leaflets. Nicotine chewing gum is helpful for some patients with health visitor anti-smoking clinics also useful.

$$\frac{6}{10}$$

Over the next year Mr Williams has several episodes of mild cardiac failure: this responds to a thiazide diuretic. He consults you as an emergency because of a two day history of a film over his (R) eye.

9.10 Discuss possible causes?

Ask *re* associated symptoms: pain and redness. History of trauma or foreign body. Change over 2 days. In absence of other symptoms and speed of onset a vascular cause seems likely.

1 Vascular (branch retinal artery thrombosis/embolus or retinal vein thrombosis), vitreous haemorrhage.
2 Retinal detachment.
3 Uveitis.   4

Far less likely.

    4 Glaucoma.
    5 Tobacco ambylopia.
    6 Cranial arteritis.
    7 Thrombocytopenia (side effect of thiazides).
    8 Brain stem lesion.   1

9.11 Outline a management plan.

Check visual acuity and fields.
Inspect outer eye.
Check fundus.
Check cardiovascular system
   including pulse and blood pressure
   ? rhythm, ? murmurs, ? thrills.
Check carotid and peripheral pulses.
Check FBC, ESR, urinalysis.
Obtain early ophthalmology opinion.

$$\frac{6}{11}$$

You now note a carotid bruit and he is commenced on aspirin. A further appointment is arranged with the cardiologist who arranges an admission for cardiac catheterization. The diagnosis of moderate aortic valve stenosis is confirmed and he is placed on the waiting list for aortic valve replacement.

9.12 Mr Williams asks you at his next appointment about the risks of cardiac surgery. How do you respond?

Explain the poor prognosis without surgery and that the only hope of cure is surgery. Reassure him that modern cardiac surgery is relatively safer but there are risks which are easily outweighed by the benefits.
Excellent results especially if weight down and non-smoker. Point out to him that he has had a number of complications although all have happily resolved.
Tell him that he is usually in hospital for around ten days and will be back at work in three months. 5

After listening to your opinion he informs you that a workmate died during this operation three years previously.

9.13 Why has he mentioned this? How do you respond?

He is scared and wonders if the same will happen to him. It is worth pointing out that techniques in cardiac surgery have improved markedly in three years and a difficult operation then could be routine now. Workmate could have been much iller than him. Point out that thousands of such operations are carried out every year and the results in the well chosen cases are excellent. Reinforce weightloss and non-smoking. Explain the risks when cardiac function severely impaired. $\frac{5}{10}$

He has an uneventful post-operative period and is discharged nine days after operation with a biological aortic valve. You are asked to visit him at the home of a lady friend. You learn from your partner that he left his wife one month before the operation.

9.14 List the problems which could result from this situation.

Doctor–patient relationship could be altered as he may be worried about your response to the situation. He could be embarrassed. However he may be unaffected and could appear normally. Surprised he had not mentioned this previously. Could be temporary arrangement and he may require accommodation and help for the future.

Break-up with wife could be related to uncertainty about operation: confidentiality is a problem. How much should his wife be told about his condition.

Is his present relationship potentially long term? 5

9.15 How do you handle the consultation?

No reference to separation unless brought up by the patient but would ask open questions so that he could talk about areas of conflict if he wanted.

You could initially introduce yourself to the lady of the house then enquire about his physical health then his social wellbeing.

An examination could be suggested and the friend asked to leave. This would give an excellent opportunity for frank discussion. $\frac{4}{9}$

You visit Mr Williams regularly over the next few weeks and he makes an excellent recovery. You are given several nice gifts over this time.

9.16 What is the significance of this?

It could be appreciation of what you have done for him but he could be seeking your approval of his new situation. It could also be a sign of insecurity on the patient's part wanting you to like him more and it may be a form of bribery. As he regards doctor as establishment figure may be seeking approval for leaving his wife.

Show your approval for the gifts but indicate firmly that this must stop. 4

9.17 Mr Williams asks you about his prognosis. How do you respond?

Excellent as long as he keeps his weight down and stays off cigarettes. Will be seen regularly in future and will require antibiotics for dentist or minor operations.

If he has told the doctor about his family situation then it is
worth pointing out that this could affect his recovery if a
sensible approach isn't followed. Also discuss his employ-
ment, exercise and sexual needs. $\frac{4}{8}$

_____

Mr Williams although better seems to be reluctant to return to work.
He informs you that his wife has commenced divorce proceedings.

9.18 What is the likely cause of his attitude?

Could be anxiety/depression related to his divorce
proceedings.
If unemployed than settlement to wife (based on last year's
earnings) likely to be less.
Could have developed cardiac neurosis.
Because of changes in social circumstances may be afraid to
meet workmates.   5

9.19 What health problems can divorce present?

Increased incidence of physical and psychiatric illness, in
particular minor physical illness/neurotic overlay.
Increased consultation rate.
Increased drug abuse, insomnia.
Increased suicide risk.
If children involved can lead to personality problems and there
can also be physically aggressive behaviour between the
couples. $\frac{6}{11}$

_____

Ten months later Mr Williams comes to see you. He is being re-
admitted to hospital for a coronary angiogram. He is asymptomatic
and wonders if this is necessary.

9.20 What do you say to him?

Admit that you are unsure yourself but assume that it is
because patients with valve problems sometimes get heart
muscle disease. This can be present without symptoms and
early detection is important.
Will 'phone cardiologist to find out more and ask him to return
in one week.   3

9.21 What is his future prognosis?

Good as long as he keeps his weight down and does not restart
  smoking. However he is still not back at work, is in the midst
  of divorce proceedings and this could be a negative factor in
  his prognosis. $\frac{3}{6}$

Commentary

On the first page the marking schedule shows the importance of the
history in general practice with 8% being given and only 6% for the
examination and investigation. On the following page 7% is
awarded for the management plan. In question 9.8 the GP is
given confidential information which has an important bearing on
the management of the patient. His skill in introducing this and
giving appropriate education is awarded highly (10%).

The differential diagnosis of the eye pathology brings 5% marks
but the examiner would give 2 marks for No 1, 1 mark each for Nos 2
and 3 and the remaining mark for any two of the uncommon causes.
This marking rewards knowledge of probability in general practice.

The latter part of the problem deals with a major life event in the
patient and a significant part of the total marks are given to problem
solving and decision making in social events where personal
attitudes play a part.

Case 10
Answers

Mary Boyle aged 33 has been a patient for 5 years. She is seen infrequently, always for self-limiting conditions. She is an unmarried secretary living with her parents in a local authority house. The family are practising Roman Catholics. She consults you one evening announcing that she is pregnant and would like you to arrange a termination.

10.1 How do you conduct this consultation?

Present a sympathetic attitude and allow time to discuss why she does want a termination? Allow her to express her feelings. Help her to consider the advantages and disadvantages of termination and continuing the pregnancy. Has she discussed it with the child's father, parents, friends or the Priest. Any prospect of marriage? Has she considered the long term consequences?

Find out basic data about pregnancy, e.g. last menstrual period.

An option to be considered would be a referral to a gynaecologist although probably not at this stage.

Assure her of confidentiality.   4

10.2 Why do you think Mary has taken such a definite attitude about pregnancy?

Shame: wishes to conceal it from parents and friends. Conflict with religious upbringing.

Circumstances of conception. Fragile relationship or transient liaison. ? Failed contraception.

Career implications. No prospect of marriage. ? Pressure for termination from child's father.

Shock: may not have considered keeping the pregnancy.

Will be poorly off financially especially if single parent.

Fear of social implications of single parenthood.

Practical housing difficulties: still lives with parents. $\frac{7}{11}$

Mary has had a relationship with a married man, a colleague at work, for the last six months. He has a young family, feels sorry about Mary's plight and is keen that she has an abortion.

10.3 What advice would you give Mary at this time?

As far as possible decide for herself as it is her baby. What is her real attitude, does she want the baby adopted? It is important that she discusses the matter with someone she can trust. Tell her that termination of pregnancy into which she feels pressurized may cause even greater guilt feelings.

Outline the practical details of termination. Reinforce the confidentiality aspect. Stress that if she has a termination she will be able to have children in the future.

Ask her to discuss the matter with you again after reflection.   4

10.4 What other agencies could help her?

You could offer to see both her and her boyfriend together but unlikely to achieve this.

Social Worker could outline support if child is born e.g. housing, child minders, DHSS allowances or adoption practicalities.

Could ask her Parish Priest to discuss it with her.

Could discuss with her family.

The health visitor would be sympathetic and offer advice and a consultant gynaecologist could also do this.

The group for single families could also offer support. $\frac{4}{8}$

You try to counsel Mary suggesting support from her family and the local Parish Priest. You arrange to see her in a week but the day before the consultation you receive a letter from the British Pregnancy Advisory Service in a town 200 miles away stating that a termination was carried out three days previously. She has been started on the 'pill'.

10.5 How do you react to this news?

Disappointed that she felt your assistance less than completely suitable. Maybe you didn't handle the consultation as well as you should.

Why did she choose this means? Has had no contact with local
 hospital and needs support.
Contact her and attempt to counsel after the event.
Future contraception will need to be discussed with her.   10

Mary arrives for her consultation the following day. How do you
conduct this?
 10.6 What advice do you give her?

No point in being aggressive. Take relaxed and friendly
 manner. Ask reasons for her decision but emphasize that she
 did not do anything wrong by consulting the BPAS. Confirm
 confidentiality. Discuss contraception: progesterone only
 pill may be best due to age but other methods should be
 mentioned.
If a smoker or overweight then requires advice about this.
Check blood pressure.
Examine her for physical complications if you feel this is
 appropriate.   5
                                                            _____
                                                                   15
                      _____

Eight days later you receive a Deputizing Service slip stating that
Mary had been seen the night before with severe chest pain:
examination was uninformative and a diagnosis of bad gastritis and
oesophagitis was made. The patient was given 100 mg pethidine
i.m. and a prescription for an antacid. No follow-up arrangements
were made.
 10.7 What would you do?

Visit at first opportunity that morning. If there is to be a delay
 then 'phone her before the surgery. Contact deputy for full
 details if slip not helpful. Find out more about the diagnosis.
 Does he often use a DDA for gastritis and oesophagitis? Does
 he not arrange a further visit in these circumstances.
When you visit you assess the need for further analgesia. Take
 a detailed history including ulcer history, dietary reason for
 gastritis, ? alcohol abuse following termination, history of
 features suggesting myocardial infarction, deep venous
 thrombosis, trauma.
Clinical examination especially chest, pulse, blood pressure,
 cardiovascular system, legs.

Depending on what has been found you may arrange an
    electrocardiogram, cardiac enzymes, chest X-ray and serum
    amylase.   6

10.8 What are the other diagnostic possibilities?

Pulmonary embolus
Myocardial infarction
Pancreatitis
Ulcer dyspepsia
Pneumonia
Spontaneous pneumothorax
Anxiety Neurosis
Other causes much less likely.   5
                                                              ──
_____   11

When you called to see her, you found her fairly comfortable. An
electrocardiogram and Chest X-ray were arranged. The latter shows
an enlarged heart with a small area of opacity in the lateral part of the
(R) mid-zone. You revisit and she is still dyspnoeic.
10.9 Give your management at this time.

Admit as emergency to general physicians or chest physicians.
    Try to reassure Mary and her family that you are taking all
    necessary steps.
Contact hospital and arrange admission. Contact ambulance
    and send letter to hospital via ambulance crew. Avoid
    conversation in house which mentioned termination of
    pregnancy but ring hospital doctor later to inform him of the
    facts.
Ask ambulance crew to give oxygen if necessary. Sedate
    adequately and again reassure patient and family that
    actions are precautionary.   4

**10.10 What explanation do you give to Mary for her
    symptoms?**

Probable small clot in lungs which could be a complication of
    recent operation. (Explain deep venous thrombosis leading
    to pulmonary embolus). Make sure family do not hear this.
Reassure her that it is likely to settle without further problems.

Is there anything she would like to ask you.

Admission is precautionary: anticoagulants are likely to be needed. Explain why. $\frac{4}{8}$

Mary makes a good recovery in hospital. She is discharged on warfarin, frusemide and a potassium supplement. You visit her at home and she asks you exactly what has been wrong with her.

10.11 What do you say?

What had she been told in hospital. Was she given an explanation of the aetiology. It is important to point out that it can also be associated with the oral contraceptive and this will be taken into account when counselled further about contraception.

Outline simply what pulmonary embolism is and why it occurred. Allow her time to express fears, frustration and any anger.

Discuss the plan for therapy in next month.

Be sympathetic and allow her to ask questions.

Reassure her that she can call you if worried.   7

10.12 What is your management plan over the next few months?

Plan follow-up counselling for psychological effects of termination. Health Visitor could be a support over this time and perhaps her Parish Priest.

Review progress of physical condition: stop potassium and when signs of congestive cardiac failure settle gradually withdraw frusemide. If she is attending hospital then should be carried out in conjunction with the hospital.

Avoid oral contraceptive and give alternative family planning advice. Encourage Mary to return to work and avoid unnecessary augmentation of the 'sick role'. $\frac{5}{12}$

Mary makes a good recovery and her therapy is gradually tailed off. She calls at the surgery four months later to inform you that she has just got engaged to an engineer who has just moved to the area. She is happy and wants to thank you for all the help you have been to her. She wonders if having a termination will reduce her chances of becoming pregnant in the future.

10.13 How do you respond to this?

Cautious reassurance that there is unlikely to be any long term
effect. Invite her to express her own thoughts and fears.
It is important at this moment to be sympathetic and to reduce
her fears although you would realize that increasing age
would decrease the likelihood of pregnancy.   4

Her fiancé does not know about her termination and she asks you
whether she should tell him.

10.14 What do you say?

What does she want to do? How close is their relationship?
Would it be affected by this? You may wish to mention the
advantages and disadvantages of doing this but the final
decision must be hers.
It would be worth pointing out that having a secret at the outset
of marriage may start things off on an unhappy footing. She
should aim to obtain his support and understanding. It may
be better that he is told now than find out later.   8
                                                              ――
                                                              12

Mary tells her fiancé about the termination and he seems to accept
this. They arrange their marriage six months ahead: they are keen to
have a family but not in the immediate future. Mary consults you
about contraceptive advice.

10.15 What do you say?

You are keen that she has satisfactory contraceptive advice but
feel the pill would not be suitable with her age and past
history of thrombo-embolic disease. IUCD is not best choice
for primigravid uterus but not absolutely contraindicated.
Increases risk of pelvic inflammatory disease.
Would an unwanted pregnancy be a disaster? Seek the views
of both Mary and her fiancé. With her religion, would she
accept other than 'natural methods'. You could describe the
rhythm and Billings method mentioning their relatively high
failure rate.
Suggest cap, diaphragm and spermicidal creams.
Give option of sheath with its drawbacks.
Having told her about all these methods, ask what she thinks.   6

10.16 What routine checks would you like to carry out?

Menstrual pattern.
Pelvic examination.
Rubella status and full blood count.
Cervical smear.
Pulse, blood pressure.
Breast examination. $\frac{5}{11}$

Mary was thrilled when she became pregnant three years later (now 39) but unfortunately had an incomplete abortion at 12 weeks followed by a dilatation and curettage.

10.17 What support could she be given at this time?

Visit from you for support. Reassure that miscarriage is not
    uncommon whether or not there has been a previous ter-
    mination. Indicate firmly that it is not a punishment.
Arrange contact with health visitor.
Arrange contact with church.   6

10.18 Outline the long term problems which she may have?

Guilt over the termination of pregnancy. She may now not
    have a family which could be a long term regret.
Could put a strain on marriage, husband who had been under-
    standing may be less so now.
Could lead to alcohol abuse by either partner or both.
Possible chance of further thromboembolic disease.
Recent events could lead to depression.
If becomes pregnant again, could have further abortion. $\frac{6}{12}$

Commentary

The MEQ about Mary Boyle is a useful test of the candidate's attitudes. On the first page the patient's attitude to termination is given 7% with the conducting of the consultation 4%. As the case develops a knowledge of the helping agencies is considered as important as the advice given to Mary. This reflects the fact that the GP is only one of many caring persons involved.

The candidate's attitudes are tested with the news that Mary has had a termination: decision making is influenced by attitudes and the mark of 10% reflects the importance. After Mary's discharge from hospital (after her pulmonary embolus) an explanation of her illness is given 7% and later when advice is sought about what she should tell her fiancé 8% is given thus reflecting the importance of the counselling role of the general practitioner.

Case 11
Answers

Mrs Jamieson, the wife of a 32-year-old dentist, telephones you at 8.30 on a Monday morning just before you are due to start surgery saying that her husband has been vomiting all night and that she would like you to call.

11.1 What factors would influence you in your response to this request?

Previous knowledge of the patient. The more familiar the more likely to go immediately.

The profession of the patient. With a doctor or dentist more than with other patients.

Knowledge of the wife. The more friendly the more likely you are to go.

Wife's attitude on the telephone. If she seems calm and capable, not upset, more likely to visit later. If anxious and agitated more likely to go immediately.

How ill is the patient? Other symptoms, e.g. chest pain, diarrhoea, blood, melaena. The more serious the symptoms the more likely you are to visit. If diarrhoea is present then a gastroenteritis might be presumed and a visit deferred or advice substituted.

Distance from the patient's house. The closer you are the more likely you are to visit quickly.

The nature of the morning surgery and the time of the first appointment, the nature of the first appointment, and the number of appointments booked. If heavily booked more likely to go early. If lightly booked more likely to wait until the end of surgery.

What does the wife want you to do?   8

When you visit you find that he is pale and ill and gives a history of central chest pain which has lasted for some four hours. Physical examination reveals a gallop rhythm, a blood pressure of 110/84 and a regular pulse with a rate of 104 per minute. You diagnose probable myocardial infarction.

11.2 What factors should you consider when deciding between home and hospital care?

Your knowledge of the studies done on home versus hospital care
The time since the onset of the infarction
The age of the patient
The general condition of the patient
Dysrhythmias
Hypotension   8
The nature of his house
The number and type of his children
Your personal availability
Availability of other members of the primary health care team
Patient's wishes
The wife's wishes
Ease of symptom control
Availability of ECG
Availability of domiciliary consultation   6
                                                                                          ──────
                                                                                              14

You decide to admit him to hospital where he is found to have had a massive anterior myocardial infarction. He has a persistent supra-ventricular tachycardia with runs of ventricular tachycardia and remains in the coronary care unit for three days. His wife asks you to visit him in hospital because he wishes to talk with you.

11.3 What are the areas that he might want to explore with you at this stage?

Prognosis:
  life
  health
Work: whether he will be able to do it again, when he will be able to return, whether it is a factor in his illness
Possible causes of his heart attack
His family and his responsibilities towards them
May feel he is not getting the plain truth from the hospital staff
May wish to discuss his will

May wish you to act as an advocate to the consultant
There are always unexpected and unknown ideas, anxieties
    and expectations   10

After a week in hospital he is discharged home on disopyramide.
He is obviously very tense and frightened and moves about his
house slowly. He has a pulse rate of 88 per minute and no abnormal
physical signs.

11.4 What problems do you now face in your management?

Psychiatric
Possibility of him becoming a cardiac cripple
Possible depressive illness and difficulties of its treatment
Anxiety state and its management
The barrier of getting him going has to be overcome   4
Physical
Use of betablocker
Use of anticoagulation
Treatment of his tachycardia
Possibility of re-infarction
Risk factors for further problems
    smoking, blood pressure, lipids, exercise, weight, glucose
        tolerance
Angina
Heart failure
Exercise tolerance
Further investigation including angiography   7
Social
Sexual activity
Sport
Alcohol
Job
Hobbies
Cannot drive in early weeks   <u>4</u>
                                                                        <u>15</u>

Two weeks after his discharge a local consultant cardiologist
telephones you to say that he is a friend of your patient and that he

would like to assess him with a view to angiography in view of the patient's age.

11.5 What factors would you take into consideration when responding to this request?

Wishes of the patient
Appropriateness of the investigation to be carried out
The feelings of the consultant physician in charge
Your experience of the cardiologist
The patient's state of mind. Could he cope with the investigation and the treatment he is on?
Anticoagulation
Patient's views about possible surgery (no point in doing angiography unless the patient will consent to surgery).   8

Three months later Mr Jamieson is still very tense and reluctant to return to work saying that he is sure that stress has contributed to his illness. He is having nightmares about the coronary care unit and has become obsessional about his weight and his eating habits.

11.6 What lines of management might be appropriate at this stage?

Referral to psychiatrist
Psychotherapy from you
Pharmacological intervention
    antidepressants (not tricyclics)
    possible use of tranquillizers
Further cardiological consultation
Either intense investigation or play down the symptoms and the seriousness of the illness   9

Two months later his wife attends with a sore throat. When leaving the consulting room she pauses at the door and asks 'Are there any tablets you can give my husband to pep up his sex drive'.

11.7 How could you respond to this?

Ask her to come back immediately to discuss the situation further

Ask to see her at a later time
Explain that medication will probably not help
Explain natural history of decreased libido in these circum-
    stances
Explore previous and immediate sexual history
Offer to see her husband to discuss the situation
Explore their non-sexual relationship
Explore her anxieties and feelings
Be optimistic and sympathetic
Offer joint consultation and consider psychotherapeutic or
    behavioural approach   13

Mr and Mrs Jamieson have four children. Richard 8, John 6,
Christopher 4, and Jenny aged 2. Mr Jamieson's mother died at the
age of 48 from a myocardial infarction. A year after Mr Jamieson's
infarction has taken place he and his wife ask you what the implications are for the children in view of the fact that their father has
had a heart attack at such a young age.

11.8 What factors would you discuss with them?

Hereditary aspects of ischaemic heart disease
Other risk factors
    familial hyperlipidaemia
    smoking
    weight
    exercise
    blood pressure
Having further children
Prospects of a continuing family history of ischaemic heart
    disease
Whether and when the children should be told
Possible value of regular surveillance   8

Eighteen months after his first infarction Mr Jamieson dies suddenly
on Christmas Eve.

**11.9 What problems will you now face in dealing with the
rest of the family subsequently?**

Bereavement syndrome with wife and with other adult
    relatives
  stunned disbelief
  anger
  depression
  acceptance   5
Probable absence of bereavement syndrome in children
Resentment of this by wife
Housing
Family income
Change in threshold for coping with physical symptoms in
    wife (especially chest pain)
Christmas will always be a vulnerable time for this family
Wife's possible increase in dependence on you to give possible
    transference
Widow's possible increased anxiety about the hereditary
    aspects of ischaemic heart disease $\underline{10}$
                                            $\underline{15}$

Commentary

The MEQ first tests a most difficult area in general practice that of deciding priorities when a number of demands are all important. The decision to send the patient to hospital or keep him at home is of the utmost importance and reflects clinical, interpersonal and social factors: the examiner's mark of 14% reflects this importance. The following question brings out the fact that the patient is always yours even when in hospital and the difficulty the GP experiences when on someone else's territory.

On Mr Jamieson's discharge from hospital high marks (15%) are awarded for a comprehensive management plan. The importance of psychiatric (obsessional state) and psychosexual aspects in the convalescence is reflected in making up 22%: these aspects bring in skills and attitudes, important areas of assessment with the MEQ.

The MEQ ends with Mr Jamieson's sudden death and the correct management at this time is reflected in the mark of 15%.

Case 12

Answers

Mrs Robertson is a 57-year-old farmer's wife who has two married daughters. She requests to be transferred to your list from that of a neighbouring doctor. There has not been a recent change of address.

12.1 What are the possible reasons for such a request?

Dissatisfaction with the other doctor
    his attitude and his manner
    his service offered e.g. length of appointment, treatment
      received
    availability: appointments system, telephone access
    his staff; possible staff change, aggressive receptionists,
      new partner
    information from District Nurses   6
Positive things about your practice
    from neighbour
    from family
    from another source
    different system of delivery of care, e.g. personal as
      opposed to mixed lists
    easier access for public transport
    possible easier car parking
    information from District Nurses   6
Patient's change in expectations
    difficult personality
    difficult illnesses
    family pressure $\frac{2}{14}$

You agree to take her on as a patient and she attends to ask for a repeat prescription for her medication for longstanding rheumatoid arthritis.

**12.2 What areas might you explore with her at this
      consultation?**

Your appointments system
Your repeat prescription system
Visiting system
Telephone access
Personal versus mixed lists
Reasons for leaving her previous doctor
Reasons for joining you
History of rheumatoid arthritis, drugs used, the complications
    and specialist advice
Other medical history
Family history
Smoking habit
Alcohol intake
Risk factors for other illness
Present problems with her rheumatoid arthritis
Expectations of treatment
Anxieties for the future
Efficacy of present treatment regime
Side effects of drugs
Hospital follow-up   12

Three months later Mrs Robertson telephones during evening surgery to request a visit because of worsening arthritis. On attending her you find her to have a hot, red, swollen left knee joint. She requests immediate private specialist advice.

12.3 What are the possible reasons for her behaviour?

Reasons for sending during evening surgery
    sudden onset of illness
    sudden loss of confidence in coping with her illness
    family pressure
    severity of symptoms
    social engagement
    previous exposure to similar problems
    an unexplored anxiety or expectation about her problem.   5
Reasons for asking for private specialist advice
    no confidence in you
    no confidence in the NHS
    realizes the implications of a sudden onset of a hot arthritis
    good experience of private medicine
    desire to make use of private health insurance
    family pressure.   5
                                           10

She is admitted to a private hospital under a consultant rheumatologist's care and is found to have a septic arthritis. After three
weeks in hospital she remains ill with a persistent septic arthritis of
both knees and of her left elbow. Her husband attends your surgery
and is clearly unhappy about the course of his wife's illness and its
treatment. He asks your advice about the best plan of action.

**12.4 What lines are now open to you? List the advantages and
disadvantages of each.**

Telephone or write to the consultant looking after Mrs
    Robertson

Advantages	*Disadvantages*
First-hand access to the facts	Possible conflict if done
Possibility of exploring the	tactlessly, both between
consultant's feelings about	the consultant and the
the case	patient, and between the
Finding out about the	consultant and you
personal relationship	
between the consultant	
and the patient and her	
husband	
Consultant's prognosis	
May precipitate a review of	
the situation by the	
consultant	

6

Arrange transfer to the National Health Service forthwith

Advantages	*Disadvantages*
Further opinion	Possible doctor/doctor
Possible more intensive	conflict
medical and nursing care	May be taking the patient
Better technical back-up	from a situation where her
It may save the patient money	problems are understood
	to one where they are not

3

Reassure all is well

Advantages	*Disadvantages*
Easy	All is probably not well and
	possible doctor/patient
	conflict or doctor/relative
	conflict

$\frac{1}{10}$

She is transferred to a National Health Service hospital under the care of a different consultant where she is found to have a septic focus in her thoracic spine with erosion of two vertebral bodies. She deteriorates rapidly and her husband requests that she be transferred home so that she may die in familiar surroundings.

12.5 What factors would influence your response to this request?

The prognosis
What is the home like
What support is available from the doctor (holiday, course of illness etc.)
What support from the primary health care team
What support from the local hospice
What support from the family
Opinion of the consultant in charge
Is the patient or her husband more likely to benefit from the transfer
The reasons for husband's request
The likely response of the husband to your reply (what does he really want)
Ease of symptom control   14

After a long and stormy illness including a major spinal operation Mrs Robertson eventually recovers and is transferred home. She has residual tinnitus caused by the powerful antibiotics which she has received. On discharge from hospital she tells you that she wishes to sue the rheumatologist who first attended her.

12.6 How might you cope with this situation?

Tell her how to complain
Tell her it is her right to complain but give her no help in doing so
Advise against complaining
Discuss the difficulties of treating her condition in the early stages
Seek advice from her second consultant
Discuss the situation with the first consultant
Ask the Medical Defence Union for advice
Seek the reasons for her dissatisfaction and attempt to difuse the situation   8

One month after his wife's discharge from hospital Mr Robertson attends with a story of sleep disturbance, anorexia and loss of concentration. He presents a picture of abject depression.

12.7 What areas might it be fruitful to explore with him at this consultation?

Guilt about the fear of his wife's death
His relationship with his wife
The relationship with the rest of his family
The success or otherwise of his farming business
His sex life
Other relationships
Drinking habit
His leisure pursuits
His ideas about his illness
His expectations about his problem
His anxieties
Any other symptoms he may have
Consider a possible organic disease as a cause of his problem   12

Three months after discharge from hospital Mr and Mrs Robertson decide to go on holiday to West Africa for convalescence.

12.8 What advice would you offer?

Holiday insurance
Immunization
Malaria prophylaxis
Adequate supply of drugs
General hygeine in tropical areas
First aid telephone number
Travel precautions
   wheelchair
   problems of a long flight with arthritis
Sunburn: possible sensitization from anti-rheumatic drugs   8

A year later Andrea Robertson, the 23-year-old married daughter of the couple who lives in another part of the country, attends your surgery and tells you that she thinks her mother and father are drinking too much.

12.9 What lines of action are open to you?

Explore the situation further with the daughter
Ignore the daughter's intervention
Send for the couple
Call on the couple
Await their next attendance
Explore their drinking habit tactfully
In the presence of a positive response offer counsel, investigation and referral (psychiatrist, counsellor, alcoholics anonymous), treatment (psychotherapy, Antabuse, admission). Give literature and arrange follow-up.
If negative reponse, consider abandoning plans ? investigate ? tackle again later.   12

Commentary

The problem starts with a patient who has changed doctor but has not changed address: this normally reflects dissatisfaction and is a difficult area for doctors to handle which is reflected in the high priority given in the marking (14%). The first consultation with a new patient is important in establishing a data base and this is given 12%.

The case develops into a number of difficult areas: firstly dissatisfaction with private care which they demanded and later seeking advice about suing a colleague. The request that Mrs Robertson should be allowed to die in familiar surroundings and the factors influencing the decision are given 14% by the examiner showing the importance of the GP in this situation.

The problem ends in another difficult situation when a daughter reports possible excess drinking in her parents and a listing of the options open score highly.

Case 13
Answers

Mr James Jones, a semi-retired gardener, aged 67, married with no children, attends the surgery with a complaint of aching pain in the left hip, of a few months duration.

13.1 What further questions would you ask of the patient?

Onset
    ? sudden
    ? any trauma
    ? gradual
Severity
    ? getting worse/staying same.
Radiation
    buttock
    knee/thigh or further.
Exacerbating features
    exercise
    rest/morning stiffness.
Relieving factors
    rest
    simple analgesics/heat
    relieved by exercise.
General health
    Specifically *re*
      Chest
      Gastro-intestinal tract
      ? Smoker.   8

13.2 What examination would you carry out?

Gait: ?limp ?using walking stick.
General appearance: Undress part being examined.
Local appearance of hip and other joints, spine.
Range of active and passive movement. ? Straight leg raising, especially internal/external rotation.

Also flexion/extension. Peripheral pulses. Reflexes if indicated
   by previous examination.
? General examination depending on findings locally.   <u>11</u>
                                                          <u>19</u>
_____

Examination reveals that movements of the left hip are restricted.
His records show that in 1975 an X-ray of cervical spine revealed
minimal spondylosis.

13.3 What further investigation would you undertake, if any?

X-ray both hips
ESR   4

13.4 What therapy would you recommend?

Explain to patient why he has pain.
Invite him to express his fears and worries. Does he want to
   know more about his condition.
Reinforce the importance of keeping mobile.
Try heat, e.g. for exacerbations.   7
Non-steroidal anti-inflammatory agent, e.g. Ibuprofen
   provided no contraindications.
± simple analgesics, e.g. Paramol (paracetamol +
   dihydrocodeine)   <u>6</u>
                                                            <u>17</u>
_____

You prescribe Ibuprofen tablets 400 mgm t.i.d. Ten days later, you
are asked to visit by his wife who is alarmed at the persistence and
severity of his pain and his threat to take an overdose of his pain-
killers. X-ray report received that morning shows minimal osteoarthritis changes in both hips with quite marked degenerative
changes in the lumbar spine.

13.5 What is your next move?

Visit
Reassessment, including history, e.g. prostatism, change in
   bowel habit, cough.
   any back trouble
   any emotional problems/symptoms of depression
   ? truly suicidal   6

Re-examination: ? any new findings + take the opportunity
    when he is in bed to examine chest and abdomen. Look
    for abdominal masses or hepatosplenomegaly,
    ?lymphadenopathy ?anaemia, cardiovascular system,
    R.S.   8
Explore both his worries and those of his wife.
Recheck FBC, ESR, Film.
Check urine for sugar and protein.
If smoker arrange a chest X-ray. $\underline{4}$

         ———————————— $\overline{18}$

On arrival at the house, you find him with continuing pain in the hip
and also in the right lower chest posteriorly attributed by him to a
recent injury.

    Chest examination revealed marked tenderness over the lower
ribs, which was the only positive finding. He appeared less well,
withdrawn and anxious but denied any suicidal threats.

13.6 What action would you take?

Increase level of analgesia: dihydrocodeine or dipipanone
Arrange for Chest X-ray and Rib X-rays. Also FBC, ESR Film,
    Urinalysis.
Again look for signs of depression
    ? marital disharmony
    ? financial worries
    ? worried *re* old age   6
Ask Mr Jones what is worrying him most.
Explore his feelings of anger, anxiety, stress and depression.
What does Mrs Jones feel about his illness, ask her to express
    her feelings.
Consider hospital admission depending on attitudes of Mr
    and Mrs Jones but the patient seems to be deteriorating
    without a diagnosis and investigations could be urgently
    required.
After discussing the problem, prescribing medication, arrange
    to revisit in 24 hours to reassess the situation. $\underline{10}$

         ———————————— $\overline{16}$

Despite reassurance and sedation he becomes increasingly tired. An
X-ray of his chest shows enlargement of the right hilum.

13.7 What is the differential diagnosis?

Bronchogenic carcinoma
Metastatic tumour
Tuberculosis
Malignant lymphoma
Sarcoidosis
Lung abscess
Aortic aneurysm
? Variant of normal.   8

Bronchial carcinoma is confirmed by subsequent hospital investigation.

13.8 How would you manage the situation?

Try and talk to wife alone about her anxieties, how much she knows, how much she thinks he should/wants to know about diagnosis. If any misunderstandings could 'phone hospital or consultant and discuss.

Explain about likely tests, alternative treatments, prognosis to her and offer support and continuity of care and reassure where possible.   10

When he is home from hospital arrange to visit him frequently and assess his situation, his fears and knowledge, how much he wants to know and remain open and available.

He will need good analgesia and here the nurse may be able to visit and help *re* future terminal care. Go for oral morphine slow release (MST) preparations, titrating the dose as necessary not forgetting laxatives to avoid constipating effects. Steroids are sometimes useful for metastases.   6

Consider with family *re* home/hospital or hospice care and encourage home care as a good alternative with support from the Health Care Team.

Make yourself available and tell family that they can call you any time. $\frac{6}{22}$

Commentary

Mr James Jones presents with a vague complaint where decisions have to be made in general practice with insufficient information. The examiner in this situation therefore considers the examination to be more important than the history. When the information from the clinical examination becomes available then the management has to be worked out. The importance of this is reflected in a mark of 13% with more than half of this being given for the explanation. The examiner is reflecting the importance of non-drug management in general practice.

The difficult situation is presented on the following page where no definite diagnosis has been made and the patient seems to be deteriorating: a logical management strategy is vital and this is reflected by the examiner giving 18% for this page. The importance of social and psychological factors is also reflected in the next page.

The final question deals with management after the bronchial carcinoma has been diagnosed and the mark of 22% reflects its breadth. The candidate has to consider the patient and his family with the question exploring attitudes towards the patient and his family.

Case 14

Answers

Mr Wilson and his wife, both aged 47, and their married son, Harold, aged 24, who lives with them, have been with the practice all their lives. Doctor–patient relationship has always been good.

Mr Wilson, who owns a garage in town, comes to see you apologizing jokingly because he has no symptoms and feels 'fit as a fiddle' and explains that he is planning to expand his business in a big way. He asks you to do a general medical check to reassure him that he is physically fit to take on the extra burden over the next few years.

14.1 What three lines of questioning would you pursue at this stage?

Was it his idea to come along or was he pushed into it by his wife? (Enquire discreetly.) If latter, maybe there is some resistance to his expanding his business in a big way.　　　3

Is this check simply to reassure him or is it for life insurance purposes? If not has he checked his policies are up-to-date and correlate with his financial plans? Also again, maybe his wife is worried about his health/plans for future. Find out about lifestyle: exercise and smoking.　　　5

Is he worried about his health for any reason (even though he says 'No'), e.g. family history of sudden death in middle age, or has he a poor history of not being able to cope with a heavy workload?

Take symptomatic enquiry ? any unreported symptoms, ? alcohol intake.　　　$\frac{4}{12}$

You agree to undertake the examination by appointment the following day.

14.2 What form do you envisage it taking?

Similar to a life insurance or pre-employment examination, e.g.
History: Systems review.
Past history: Operations, etc.

Social: Alcohol, cigarettes, drugs.
Examination
  Weight, Height, Eyes, ENT, Lungs, cardiovascular
    system (blood pressure), Abdomen (Urine for sugar,
    protein). Brief CNS, rectal examination, chest X-ray or
    electrocardiogram if appropriate.   6

Physical examination of Mr Wilson the following day is negative. As
he is dressing he says 'Good for another thirty years then, Doc?'
  14.3 What do you reply?

  Try to make his optimism more realistic by being honest and
    saying, 'Well, of course routine physical examinations at
    your age do not usually turn up much and in some surveys
    is not thought to be cost effective. I can say you are in good
    health now, however cannot predict into the future. Despite
    this there is nothing to stop you from going ahead with your
    plans but you should look after yourself.'
  Mention importance of not smoking and drinking in
    moderation in relation to being healthy.   8
                                                              ———
                                                                   14

A week later during morning surgery the Casualty Officer at the
Infirmary telephones to say that Mr Wilson has collapsed at his
garage and had just been brought in dead to the Infirmary. He asks if
you would be prepared to issue a death certificate.
  14.4 How do you reply?

  (Surprised and shaken inwardly), enquire as to whether there
    were any witnesses present when he collapsed, i.e. was it a
    natural death, also what was the description of the mode of
    death, e.g. like a myocardial infarction or was it something
    unusual, e.g. a fit.   5
  Obviously if any suspicious circumstances consider a
    Coroner's case (or Procurator Fiscal) but most likely this was
    a myocardial infarction and as you saw him within 14 days of
    death you can sign the certificate and after discussing the
    details with the Casualty Officer probably would say Yes.
    However, you'd probably be happier with a post mortem
    examination. You are not obliged to see the body but should
    and would do so as part of etiquette. Also most likely the
    relatives will be there and needing some sympathy and

support from their GP. When visiting the hospital to see the body you could find out from the Casualty Officer how the family have reacted to the sudden death. $\frac{7}{12}$

You suspect that Mr Wilson has died from a coronary thrombosis because of the further details of the 'collapse' given to you by the Casualty Officer.

14.5 Name five 'high risk' factors in the aetiology of coronary artery disease in young men.

1. Smoking: incidence twice as high in smokers than non-smokers.
2. Hypertension: Framingham study presence of mild hypertension increases risk of fatal coronary threefold.
3. Hyperlipidaemia: risk slightly increased at low levels, i.e. just above upper limit of normal, but sharp rise at upper levels.
4. Positive family history.
5. Diabetes mellitus: coronary heart disease now commonest cause of death in adult diabetes.   10

You decide to visit Mrs Wilson after lunch and anticipate a difficult consultation.

14.6 What are the three recognized stages of the grief reaction?

Beginning. Can last hours or days. Feelings of numbness are interspersed with outbursts of anger and distress.

Middle. Period of 'painful pining' which is accompanied by memories of the events that led up to the death. There is a strong feeling of the presence of the dead person. Person afraid of impending madness and requires reassurance. May be afraid to mention this. May diminish in intensity in week or two. A scapegoat may be sought and the medical profession are often criticized. Undue feelings of guilt require special help.

Final. Lasts about a year and consists of apathy, depression and aimlessness. Taking up a new activity may be a help. By end of second year, it is normal for life to be reorganized.   10

On a follow-up visit to Mrs Wilson three days later, the son, Harold, is present and they jointly accuse you of negligence because you had declared Mr Wilson healthy following the examination a week prior to his death. They declare their intention to report you to the 'authorities' to protect other people from your incompetence.

14.7 How do you reply?

That you sympathize with their feelings and are aware of how they must feel. Allow them to express feelings of anger, grief, anxiety and stress. Point out that a thorough physical examination seldom uncovers coronary heart disease and cannot predict a sudden coronary and that you wish you could have. A sudden death is one of the most poorly understood areas in medicine even in the areas of the Health Service where high technology is the normal means of monitoring. Unfortunately doctors cannot forecast such events.   8

Do not go on the defensive too much nor try to get into arguments about details as their hostility to the doctor is fairly typical of a grief reaction. The right idea is to remain available and open for discussion, sympathetic and not to 'run away'.

Offer support and follow-up. Ask whether they wish you to return or whether they would prefer to be left alone.   8
                                                                        ──
                                                                        16

Mrs Wilson comes to the surgery a week later asking you to forgive her for being too hasty. You wonder if she may be depressed.

14.8 Name five symptoms or signs which would help support a diagnosis of depression associated with the grief reaction.

1 Sleep disturbance, early morning wakening.
2 Weight loss and loss of appetite.
3 Suicidal ideations; Hallucinations and visions of deceased.
4 Protracted guilt/hostility/crying.
5 Loss of concentration, lack of energy/apathy/self neglect.   10

Two weeks later Harold Wilson comes to the surgery complaining of chest pains on exertion and demands to see a heart specialist.

14.9 How would you handle this situation?

Take a formal history of exacerbating factors, relieving factors, radiation of pain, etc. ? Smokes.

Do a routine physical: blood pressure, heart, lungs. 4

Discuss the problem and purposely direct the consultation towards the bereavement, how he is coping: sleep, appetite, work, has he cried, what are his anxieties, i.e. generally explore in a counselling fashion his psychological problems 6

Explain to him he is unlikely at his age to have heart problems and reassure. However be open to referring him if he persists in his request, and probably do an electrocardiogram. With a good relationship there should be less necessity to refer and he will feel better with sympathy, support and continuity of care.

However if he persists and in view of what happened to father may be wiser to refer him to specialist. 6

—

16

Commentary

The MEQ about Mr Harold Wilson specifically tests knowledge on three separate pages: this is more than usual in this type of question. In question 14.5 five high risk factors are sought, in 14.6 the three stages of the grief reaction and in 14.8 the symptoms and signs of depression: these parts make up 30% of the marks despite taking up a larger proportion of the problem reflecting the greater importance of skills and attitudes in the MEQ. This is also shown in 14.2 and 14.3 where the explanation to Mr Wilson is given a higher mark than the detail of the physical check-up.

One-third of the marks are given in two pages of the problem; question 14.7 when the doctor is in an impossible situation with his competence being called into question and his attitude to his patient is being tested: question 14.9 when the son presents with symptoms related to the condition which caused the father's death. This tests decision making and attitudes to the patient and other members of his family.

Case 15

Answers

Mr and Mrs Patel are an Asian couple in their forties with three children from 3–13 years. Mr Patel works as a waiter in a local Indian restaurant. He came to the surgery one evening and says he has felt very tired and weak for several months.

15.1 How would you assess the significance of this complaint?

History

Present problem, how long: features, description, time of day, associated phenomena.

His explanation of the cause.   3

Brief systemic history looking especially for symptoms suggestive of organic disease, e.g. short of breath, swelling of ankle, chest and abdominal pain, diarrhoea, severe headache, backache etc.

Past history, family history, job history, financial/ accommodation.   2

Examination

Looking especially for anaemia, cardiovascular system abnormalities, abdominal tenderness, papilloedema and test urine.   2

Consider *investigation* but only chest X-ray and FBC at this point. $\underline{2}$

                                         $\underline{9}$

You find nothing abnormal on examination and then he reveals that the weakness occurs after attempting intercourse.

15.2 Why do you think he presented the problem as he did?

Embarrassed, shy, timid.   3

Didn't know how to present the problem/didn't recognize connection.   2

Language, class, culture barrier.   2

Hoping for medicine without revealing the problem.	2
Assessing the doctor to see if he/she was sympathetic to 'real' cause.	2
	11

You do not find it easy to help Mr Patel and ask him and his wife together. At the next consultation, Mrs Patel does not come but a cousin comes, she says, 'as an interpreter'.

15.3 Why is this and what does it mean?

Mrs Patel couldn't come, language barrier, too many children and no one to leave them with, is not well. Mr Patel refuses to let his wife come.	3
Cultural, religious, social difficulties.	2
Pressure not to divulge interpersonal stress within or outside family.	2
Confusion over what doctor intended.	2
Cousin acts as 'mediator'.	2
	11

Some months later Mrs Patel brings their youngest child aged 3 years and says that he always has 'coughs and colds' and occasional 'noises in the chest'. She asks for 'strong medicine' because he is keeping everyone awake at night.

15.4 How might a GP respond to her request?

Sympathy/empathy.	2
History, especially of asthma, eczema, hay fever. History of present problem: URTI's cough, and 'noises'. General build and development.	2
Examination especially height, weight, respiratory system, ear, nose and throat and skin.	2
Possible investigations	
Chest X-ray	
FBC	
Allergy tests.	2

Plan
    Explain/explore
    Prescribe
    Counsel
    Primary Health Care Team
    Follow-up. $\frac{3}{11}$

Ramesh is thought to have asthma and settles quite well on oral medication. Some weeks later Mr Patel telephones and asks for a second opinion about Ramesh as his employer has recommended him to consult a local private practitioner.

15.5 How could you deal with this problem?

Immediate
    Ask Mr Patel to bring in Ramesh again to the surgery and
        you'll discuss it.   2
At this consultation ask
    Why his employer felt he should have a second opinion?
    What did he (Mr Patel) and his wife think of this idea?
    Had there been any changes in the past few weeks?
    Examine.   3
Options
    Yes
    No
    Possible? $\frac{2}{7}$

A few months later Mr Patel contacts you again on the telephone and asks you to see his father who has recently arrived from India. He says his father has had diarrhoea for weeks.

15.6 What might be the cause of his complaint and how should it be managed?

Cause of diarrhoea
    Infective
    Viral: enteroviruses.
    Bacterial: typical paratyphoid, salmonella, shigella,
        cholera.   3

Parasitic: amoebic dysentery, giardia lamblia, worms of
   various kinds, schistosomiasias.
Toxic: staphylococcal.
Non-infective: diverticulitis, colitis, enteritis due to
   inflammation of bowel, carcinoma, IBS.   1
Management depends on aetiology, local and general hygiene
   important.   2
                                                                        ――
                                                                        6

Investigation of Mr Patel's father reveals hookworm and he is given
treatment which successfully clears his symptoms. However he
appears in the surgery a month later with his son and asks for a
tonic.

15.7 How would you handle this request?

Explore
   First ask him why he wants a tonic? Did he or someone else
      in the family suggest it, i.e. expectations and his view
      (and son's).   3
   History. General health especially appetite. Indigestion,
      stool frequency, colour and consistency, any blood in
      stools? Significant past history, i.e. previous illnesses.
      Drugs/alcohol/smoking. Job in India.   3
   Examination. Especially gastrointestinal tract but also look
      for fever, anaemia, glandular enlargement,
      splenomegaly and hepatomegaly.   2
   Investigation. Possible further stool samples to confirm
      clearance, Hb, biochem screen.   1

Options
   Prescribe tonic or similar.
   Refuse point blank.
   Discuss pros and cons of giving tonic taking the patient's
      view into consideration and prescribe if necessary.   2
   Follow up important.
   Throughout offer sympathy and empathy.   ――
                                                                        11

Some months later Sabina, the Patel's elder daughter now aged 16 years, consults at the surgery with headaches and panic feelings which she has difficulty in controlling.

15.8 What might cause these symptoms and how would you initially manage the problem?

Organic
　Thyrotoxicosis
　Brain tumour
　Sinus problems.   2
Non-organic
　Tension headaches
　Migraine
　Premenstrual tension
　Anxiety/depression
　Situation of home/school/relationships.   3
History
　Describe headache, where, frequency, type, duration,
　　associated features? General health, weight loss,
　　vomiting, diarrhoea, blurred vision, other central nervous
　　system symptoms, ear, nose and throat symptoms or pain. 3
Examination
　Especially central nervous system, and ear, nose and throat,
　　also blood pressure.
　Also origins of depression/anxiety.   2
Investigation
　Hb/Chest and skull X-rays/T4.   1
                                                                      ——
                                                                       11

Tests reveal thyrotoxicosis and she is treated with carbimazole but she feels she is unable to take her 'O' level examinations. Mr and Mrs Patel ask for your help.

15.9 Is there anything you can do about this and does your action have any disadvantages?

You can write to the 'O' Level Examination Board and explain
　the circumstances. They may arrange a special examination
　or sometimes to award the result on the basis of in-course
　work.   3

Or you can suggest to Sabina to take the examination and at
    the same time you could write to the Examining Board so
    that the medical situation is considered by the Examiner.   3
Or you can suggest to Sabina to get on and take another
    examination.   1
Or you can suggest to Sabina to miss the examination and take
    it again later.   1
Or you can ask Sabina to discuss the pros and cons of the
    various options.   1
The first four options do not necessarily involve Sabina in
    making a decision and the other does and it is desirable that
    she is involved. $\underline{2}$
                      $\underline{\underline{11}}$

**15.10 What do you know about the way Asian families are
organized, and could you and your Primary Care Team
anticipate any problems and handle them better in the
future?**

That Asian families may not present their illness in the same
    way as European families.   3
That relationships within the family are often different, several
    generations/siblings/cousins/in-laws living together.
Motivation for upward social and educational mobility is high.
Education and training is encouraged.   3
Tolerance, acceptance, exchange, knowledge,
    understanding.   2
Learn language, culture, ultimately religion.
Consider Asian health care worker.   2
Consider leaflets in Hindi, etc.
Consider good relationships. $\underline{2}$
                      $\underline{\underline{12}}$

Commentary

In the MEQ about the Patel family question 15.2, seeking the
candidate's range of options about why the patient presented as he
did, is given 11% but the first question about history, examination
and investigation only scored 9%. This reflects the importance of
testing the candidate's thought processes. In question 15.4 being
empathic to the patient's request is considered by the examiner as
important as either the history or the physical examination.

The low priority given to knowledge in the MEQ is shown in question 15.6 when only 4 marks are given for the causes of diarrhoea. In question 15.7 exploration of the request with consideration of the options scores almost half of the marks available for that particular page: this is testing the candidate's thought process before coming to a specific decision.

In question 15.8, when the candidate is asked the causes of 'headaches and panic feelings', the examiner reflects the importance of probability in general practice with 3% being given for nonorganic causes and only 2% for organic. At the section on the 'O' levels a mark of 11% is given for problem solving, considering the available options and making an appropriate choice. 12% is given for the final question which tests the candidate's knowledge of immigrants and their management in general practice.

Case 16

Answers

Harry and Gertrude Marcus live with their son Robert, aged 17 years, and daughter Tracy, aged 15 years, in a thirties semidetached suburban house. Mrs Marcus' mother, aged 79 years, also lives with them. In early Spring one year Mrs Marcus, now aged 44 years, comes to the surgery complaining of heavy prolonged periods and depression.

16.1 What might be the cause of her symptoms? Outline your management.

Gynaecological problems
Menorrhagia, polymenorrhea of hormonal origin
Fibroids
Pelvic infection
Menopause   2
Emotional/psychological/family problems
Relationship/problems: husband–wife, grandparents,
        parents, children
Depression ± anxiety
Financial problems
Others   2
Management
History: gravida, length of periods, cycle, how heavy,
        accompanying pain, clots, functional disturbance   2
Examination: general, especially blood pressure, urine,
        breasts, pelvic speculum and bimanual   1
Investigations: Hb, vaginal smear, cervical smear
        hormone levels including T_4 1
Plan:
    Discuss options: what does patient want?
    Prescribe progesterone latter half of cycle or combined pill
        (less safe).   2
                                                                      ___
Refer to gynaecologists for dilatation and curettage.
                                                                      10

Gertrude settles well on progesterone in the second half of the menstrual cycle. A few weeks later Harry comes to see you very upset. He says his mother-in-law is seeing things and talking to herself and really feels it is about time she went somewhere permanently.

16.2 How would you handle this request?

Explore possible causes

Empathy/sympathy with him and problems	2
History from Harry of mother-in-law's health and family in general	2
See mother-in-law and take history/examine/investigate	2
View of herself and family on options for future	2

Options for management

Treat any condition revealed by examination
Consider use of support, i.e. (Primary Care Team)
Refer to geriatrician or psychogeriatrician or psychiatrist
See again next week—no specific decision
Day centre/day hospital, i.e. day care
Short term admission
  GP Unit

geriatrician or psychogeriatrician	3
	11

Grandmother's chest infection improves and with it her mental state, but Harry sees you two or three times in a few weeks complaining of indigestion. You find nothing abnormal on examination, but antacids do not appear to help.

16.3 What are your management options and what are their advantages and disadvantages?

Detailed history of indigestion

Further history: length of symptoms, time of day, how long it lasts, vomiting, diarrhoea, colour of stools, general health especially weight, appetite and digestion.	2

Options	Advantages	Disadvantages	
Rest and continue antacids	Safe. May be effective. Break from work.	May not work. Loss time off work.	2

Trial of H$_2$ antagonist	Effective. Does not involve specialist referral or time off work.	May mask carcinoma. Not desirable without endoscopy.	2
Refer for endoscopy	Definitive diagnosis may be made or refuted.	Uncomfortable. Only show stomach and duodenum. Time off work.	2
Refer for barium meal	Diagnosis made or refuted but less effective than endoscopy.	Less effective than endoscopy. Expose to X-rays.	1
Refer to specialist physician	Specialist will sort problem out. Patient and family may be pleased.	Loss of care of patient. Anxiety by patient and family. Expensive use of resources.	1
			10

Harry's symptoms settle on a course of cimetidine after a negative endoscopy but the same month Tracy consults because of 'terrible spots'. You can see a few acniform spots. She asks for hormone treatment 'because it helped a friend and also because I have bad periods'.

16.4 Outline what you could do to help Tracy and what you might actually do?

Agree with her and prescribe hormone treatment.
Refuse point blank. 2
Negotiate
  Find out why she feels her acne is so bad and more about her 'bad periods'. What is 'bad' about them? Ask gently about boy friends and whether she is asking indirectly for a contraceptive pill. 2
Consider general history and examination
  History:
    acne, periods, significant PH and FH
    social functions, school/friends/parents/sexuality. 2

Examination of blood pressure, urine, skin, gynaecological
   CS/PV if appropriate.
Preferably negotiate and examine Tracy appropriately
followed by discussion of problems, prescribing simple
therapy with few side effects first unless she has already
tried them.   2
Local creams
Ultraviolet light
Oxytetracycline/erythromycin before hormonal treatment
   unless she should in your view take a contraceptive pill
   (she is only 15). $\frac{2}{10}$

Much to your surprise only the following week Harry comes to the
surgery with Gertrude and tells you of Robert's abnormal
behaviour. He shouts, argues and locks himself in his room. They
ask you to come round right away, but agree to postpone the visit till
the end of the surgery.

16.5 What possible causes may there be for this problem and how could you separate them?

Causes
Illness
   physical: encephalitis, brain tumour
   marital: anxiety, psychosis   2
Personal psychological/emotional problems
   Drugs, alcohol
   Personal crisis:
     relationships
     problems at college/work   2
Family Pressures
   stress/conflict
   Robert is suffering for the rest of the family   2
Explore
See Robert and explore physical/mental/personal history
Exclude psychosis/anxiety and depression
See rest of family for exploration.   2
Management
Calm, relaxed approach

Options
  Robert's
  Family's
  Yours
Follow-up/accessibility
Prescribe
Refer to Primary Care Team.   2
                                                              ────
                                                                10
                  ───────────────

When you arrive Robert is locked in his room and a record player is blaring noisily; conversation with Robert is impossible but Harry offers to break down the door so you can get in and 'deal' with the situation.

16.6 Do you agree or not and what are the implications of each move you can make?

	Positive implications	*Negative implications*
Agree	Immediate solution to problem you 'find out what is going on'.	Anger between father and son may lead to fight and injury.
	Instant action.	Emotions very high.
	Problem is over today.	Damage to door/ house.
		Have not established adequate reasons for this action. Robert not involved in decision. 2
Refuse	Robert may be pleased.	Harry may be angry with you.
	Chance for emotions to calm down.	Not an 'easy' solution now.
	Opportunity for calm, rational approach.	More time and 'lost' to doctor.
	Opportunity for obtaining help as necessary.	Emotions remain changed.
		2

Negotiate	*With Robert*		
	Involves him in decisions.	May be very time consuming. May have to be conducted through a locked door.	
	Opportunity for acceptance of his angers/fears/ anxieties/ problems.	Loss of control by doctor.	
		Family not in control either.	2
	With Harry and the rest of the family		
	May allow a calm relaxed approach by them.	They may not be enthusiastic. You may be abused.	
	Problems may be partially alleviated.	Time consuming.	2
Wait and review	Allow tempers to cool.	Time consuming. No decision made.	
	Problems may be resolved within family.		2
			10

Robert is thought to have been abusing soft drugs and agrees to a period of inpatient care in the local psychiatric hospital. The Psychiatrist would like to offer some family therapy and asks your help and assistance. The family in their turn also come and ask you what this therapy is and what Robert's problem has to do with them.
16.7 How do you respond?

What is family therapy
Involvement of whole family in discussion of difficulties/ problem with Psychiatrist/Psychotherapist/Psychologist.   3
Continued process of therapy approximately once a week for a period of time: exploring feelings and attitudes of the family as a unit.   2
What have Robert's problems to do with the family
His problems could be caused by family stresses and strains so help for family may help him, i.e. he is the sign of family stress.   2

Help for Robert may be enhanced by reducing family stress. $\dfrac{2}{9}$

_____

Family therapy does not really succeed and after some weeks Robert leaves hospital and goes to a hostel but does not settle very well and returns home periodically and causes much friction. Late one Saturday night when you are on duty there is an emergency request for a visit to the Marcus household. The call comes from Gertrude who says that Harry and Robert are fighting and 'you must come quickly doctor or he'll kill him'. She rings off.

16.8 What could you do now and why?

Go immediately and face the difficulties you will find.
   Problem then will be dealt with and some anxieties reduced.   2
Do not bother.
Telephone deputizing service or police.
   The former is understandable but not desirable. The latter
     may be sensible as long as you also go yourself.   2
Ask police to accompany you.
   They may help you to diffuse the situation but their
     presence may sometimes aggravate the tension.   2
Ask the local authority social worker to go with you.
   Presence of a third or fourth involved party is often of great
     value in calming things down and working out practical
     solution.   2
On arrival
Be calm, even if situation at the home is not calm.
Listen and explore with all present.
Decide what happens to-night to Robert. Where does he stay,
   at home or relative/friend/neighbour/elsewhere.
To-morrow you can try to sort things out better. $\dfrac{2}{10}$

_____

With the aid of neighbours and the police the fight is ended and Harry and Robert's superficial wounds are cleaned and dressed. Harry says he's got 'to get Robert out of the house', Gertrude is crying, mother is asleep upstairs and Tracy is out. Robert says he

didn't start it. You find Robert has formally left the hostel and has
been staying at home or sleeping rough.

16.9 How do you handle this current situation?

Difficulties you face
Physical injury.
No easy solution to cause of fight.
Is Robert psychiatrically ill or back on drugs or is this a family
    crisis?
Where does Robert go to-night?   2
Options
Robert stays at home to-night—but fighting may occur again.
Robert stays with relatives/neighbours/friends to-night and
    we try to sort things out more calmly to-morrow.
Robert goes elsewhere? back to hostel/hostel for homeless/
    hospital etc.   2
Immediate i.e. to-night
Calm relaxed approach essential even if situation at home is
    not calm.
Listen, ask, explore.
Decide what to do to-night—then leave rest open.   2
To-morrow
Consider next options with Robert and family hopefully now
    more calm.
Does Robert stay at home or not—and if not, where does he
    go?
Consider enlisting help of psychiatrist/psychotherapist/
    psychologist who saw Robert and family before.   2
Long-term: within a few days/weeks
See Robert (if appropriate) and family approximately weekly
    to follow progress and offer help to avoid further conflict
    and to assist in rehabilitation. $\frac{2}{10}$

After years of infrequent consultation, you find on review that this
family have generated about 20 consultations and 8 visits in a year.

**16.10 Why should this be and what, if anything, could have
      been done earlier to prevent these problems arising?**

Causes of recent 'illhealth'

Grandmother's increasing dependence.   2

Family relationships strained
    husband–wife
    grandmother–daughter
    grandmother–son-in-law
    grandmother–grandchildren
    parents–children   2

Identity crisis for adolescents.

Alcohol and drug abuse.

Cramped accommodation especially felt by adolescents.

Financial difficulties/job/problems, especially as Harry has four
    dependents to maintain.

Genuine physical and mental illness causing stress.   2

Prevention

Regular review of grandmother's state of physical and mental
    health including district nurse/health visitor.   2

'Better care' at crisis including whole family.

Use of Primary Care Teams especially psychologist/social
    worker/counsellor if available.

Earlier referral for special help.

                                                     $\overline{10}$

Commentary

The MEQ about the Marcus family is very complex and presents situations where it is difficult to give a solution. Three generations in the family live together and the problem starts with Mrs Marcus presenting with two complaints which have some overlap. The husband then calls to report strange symptoms in his mother-in-law: exploration of the possible causes is given 8% by the examiner with the options for management being given a lower priority.

The importance of problem solving in the MEQ is reflected by the examiner in questions 16.3 and 16.6 where the candidate is asked for options, implications and choices firstly with Harry's indigestion and secondly when Harry wants you to 'deal with the situation'. A maximum of 10% can be scored on each page. When Tracy presents in question 16.4 with her 'bad spots' 4% is given for the part handling her request reflecting the importance in general practice of explanation. When the son behaves abnormally the examiner awards 8% for the consideration of aetiological factors bringing out the importance of psychological factors in primary care. Later in the problem when violence develops the doctor is presented with an impossible situation and tests his decision making in this context e.g. ? to involve police.

The doctor's attitude to the patient and his family is tested in question 16.9 and the case ends by asking the candidate to consider the options open to him in a high demand family.

Case 17

Answers

Thomas is a bachelor of 61 years of age, and a railway engine driver, who has been found to be suffering from cervical spondylosis, severe enough to give him temporary obstruction to cerebral blood flow on sudden neck movements. He also has peptic ulceration and mild hypertension. He has now been off work for several weeks, because of his cervical spondylosis, and is now thinking about returning to work. He comes to tell you that he has to see the 'Railway Doctor', and wants to know what will happen about his work.

17.1 What do you say to him?

Explanation of why he has to see the doctor employed by the
  railway.
 need to assess him after a period off work
 need to assess if he can still perform his duties.   3
Employing authority's medical adviser can only have access to
  GP's records with patient's written permission.   1
Explore patient's own attitude to his work and his fitness to do
  it.
 responsible position as a driver
 can he cope with his disability and his work.   3
Pave the way for the likelihood of
 alternative employment in the railway
 early retirement
 employment outwith the railway. $\frac{3}{10}$

Thomas gets back to work and apart from coping quite well with his work, he has a vagotomy and pyloroplasty for a haematemesis from his duodenal ulcer. For 3 years remains quite well, until he begins to complain of dragging in his legs when walking.

The neurologist to whom you refer him is surprised that he is still working, and thinks Thomas may have had some brain stem infarct, and perhaps further cerebral ischaemic episodes.

He is, at last, deemed unfit to work, and given early retirement. He announces that he will be going to stay with his fiancée of many years, who has said she will look after him.

17.2 What problems do you see in the immediate period, and the future for Thomas?

Medical and psychiatric problems
    Progressive disablement 2
    Loss of independence and having to depend on others 1
    Lowering of morale, depression 2
    Frustration at not being able to work 1
    May be other pathology developing since the neurologist
      was vague. 1
Social problems
    Financial: if retired on health grounds, his work pension
      may be updated to full amount 2
    Not yet eligible for OAP 1
    Living with fiancée: he may be better looked after, but it may
      be a strain on the relationship if she doesn't realize the
      extent of his disability 2
    Decreasing mobility 1
    Isolation from the community if unable to get out. 1

                                                  14

Two years later, after myocardial infarction, he is admitted to hospital following an overdose of Ibuprofen and alcohol. The Ibuprofen had been prescribed to help his neck and back pain. He is again referred to a neurologist, by the physicians but he sends for a home visit because he has never received his neurology appointment, and you notice the address you are requested to visit is that of his fiancée, and not that on his medical record.

17.3 How do you cope with the situation?

    Acceptance of request for house call, although inappropriate
      request.
      Modification of GP's reaction because of knowledge of
        Thomas's mental state. 2

On arrival check if he has notified the hospital of change of
    address.
  It is the patient's responsibility to notify change.
  Check the stability of his location.   1
Notify hospital yourself of change of address and ask for
    another appointment to be forwarded.   1
Discuss reasons for his overdose
  serious
  accidental
  crisis   2
  pain
  alcohol excess—try to gently explore
  depression—assess mental state now
  ? need for psychiatric referral   4
Discuss with fiancée the danger of alcohol and tablets.   1
Assess how they are getting on. Is she finding it too much?   1
                                           12

His fiancée thinks he should be admitted again, particularly as she is
soon going to be admitted herself to hospital for a hysterectomy.
Thomas is just sitting in a chair, looking rather down-in-the-mouth,
and there is a smell of urine in the room. His fiancée, who seems to
dominate him, tells you that he is often unable to get to the toilet and
asks if the nurse could come in to help him.

**17.4 What problems do you see arising now, and how would
you cope with them?**

Fiancée's health
  Not your patient, but would help to know whether the
    hysterectomy is for a benign or malignant lesion.
  How long will she be unfit to cope with him.   3
Fiancée's attitude
  Is the apparent domination real.
  Is she being mis-guided in not letting him do more for
    himself.   1
Smell of urine
  Mention this, with a risk of upsetting either party.   1
  Explore reasons (physical) Urinary tract infection (dip
    slide—microscopy).
  Could use collection of specimen as excuse to get nurse to
    call to assess situation and placate fiancée.   3

Abdominal examination.
? per rectum may be difficult.
Mental, i.e. just forgets.
Check drug therapy as a cause, e.g. diuretics.   3
Discuss the possibility of Thomas coping on his own if fiancée
   is in hospital. As this seems unlikely, assure fiancée you
   will look into the possibility of some form of inpatient
   care.   2
Discuss with practice team. $\underline{1}$
   $\overline{14}$

After pressing for admission for the period while his fiancée is in
hospital, and to get him assessed further neurologically, the consultant returns him to your care, with a diagnosis of brain stem
vascular disease and cerebral atrophy, with a further comment,
'Perhaps you would arrange for geriatric supervision for this man
now that he is within their age group'. You note he is indeed now 65.

17.5 How would you react to this request?

Own feelings
   annoyance at geriatric assessment not having been arranged
     while in hospital
   'Well it's my job anyway'
   Neurologist has washed his hands of the case and has
     passed it back
   Now duty bound to ask for a geriatric assessment to make
     sure 'everything' has been done   3
Discuss with health care team
   Health Visitor
   Nurse
   Social Worker   2
Geriatric Assessment
   Out-patient: limitation as will not assess him in his house
   Domiciliary visit probably more appropriate   2
Risk of something happening if one delays in seeking geriatric
   assessment $\underline{1}$
   $\overline{8}$

The geriatrician who does the domiciliary visit is not too thrilled at
the idea of Thomas being landed on his plate, especially in view of
his urinary incontinence which is deemed to be due to prostatism,
and suggests that now that his fiancée is home, all effort should be

made to manage him in the community, even although he acknowledges he is walking with a shuffling gait now, and may be difficult.

You are awaiting a urology opinion on Thomas anyway regarding his prostate.

17.6 What agencies can you contact and how can they help to maintain Thomas in the community?

Own Practice Team
  health visitor
    advice on general services and allowances
  nurse
    discuss general care and in particular his urinary problem
    ? a catheter while awaiting operation
    risk of infection
    might be easier to manage
    aids: Zimmer or stick
  social worker:
    allowances (attendance, mobility)   5
Domiciliary Physiotherapy, if available to keep up mobility.   1
Occupational Therapist
  aids in the house
  bathing aids.   1
Home Help probably not given when fiancée is at home.   1
Voluntary Agencies to relieve fiancée.   1
Press for Geriatric Day Care.   <u>1</u>
                                                                                              <u>10</u>

Eventually, Thomas has a transurethral prostatectomy, but is sent home with an indwelling catheter because he cannot control his bladder. You persuade the geriatrician to take him to Day Hospital twice a week, on a Tuesday and Friday, for physiotherapy and to relieve the burden at home. He has had a fair bit of discomfort from the catheter, but your nursing sister is quite happy about things.

At 5.50 pm one Friday evening, his fiancée 'phones to say he has just returned from Day Hospital in great pain from his catheter. She has 'phoned the Day Hospital to complain about him being sent home, and says the ambulance men who brought him home say he should never have been allowed home. She tells you to call that night and admit him to hospital.

17.7 How do you feel, and what can you do?

Frustration
    late call for no great reason as would presumably not have
        been sent home from Day Hospital if ill, may not have
        reported discomfort at Day Hospital.   1
Disbelief that ambulance men would say such a thing.   1
Feeling of being manipulated by fiancée, and resentment at
    being 'told' to call.   1
Talk to fiancée, on the 'phone, but probably will not achieve
    much.   1
    Check with Day Hospital (if personnel still there) on his
        condition.   1
Bottle up anger and go to see him to assess his discomfort.
    if necessary refer for urological opinion
    or change catheter yourself
    or ask for bladder lavage by nurse.   2
Avoid confrontation with fiancée. $\frac{1}{8}$

A few weeks later, the geriatrician 'phones you to say he is fed up with Thomas's fiancée interfering so much, and playing off one service against the other. He says he has heard that she has complained to the local district councillor about the lack of care given to Thomas, but no official complaint has yet been received. However, in view of this, he suggests admitting Thomas for an independent assessment in hospital as to his capabilities, as he feels he could do much more for himself.

17.8 What skills would be assessed, and by whom, and how would this admission help the situation?

Mobility, by physiotherapist and doctor.   1
Skills for day-to-day living
    dressing, by occupational therapist
    bathing, by nurse
    cooking, by occupational therapist
    ability to handle finance, by social worker.   4
This admission would relieve tension all round and give a fair
    chance to assess Thomas without his fiancée interfering. If
    successful, it would help Thomas to re-establish his morale
    and independence and make him realize what he could do
    for himself. His fianceé would also get a break for a while.   6
One would also have evidence if a complaint surfaced. $\frac{1}{12}$

Thomas is found to be continent, happy, able to manage dressing and caring for himself in every way except cooking. A case conference is called and after discussion, it is decided that he could manage fairly well on his own at his own home with the long term possibility of admission to a residential home for the elderly, provided he remains continent. Thomas is perfectly willing to entertain the idea of a residential home, and his fiancée is called in to the case conference to be told of the decision. It is decided that as you are attending the case conference as Thomas's GP, and you know the fiancée as well, although she is not a patient of yours you should be the spokesman for the group.

17.9 What would you say to her, and what do you think briefly would be the outcome of this?

Initially reassure her that this was not the team and Thomas versus her. 2

Explain the outcome of the assessment and explain that when having to cope on his own, he can manage to carry out most day-to-day functions such as dressing, emptying his catheter bag, walking to the toilet and washing himself. The only thing is that he cannot cook for himself. She should continue to encourage him to do these things and perhaps tell her that she is going to have to be 'cruel' to be kind. It is not in Thomas's best interest if she does everything for him. He has indicated that he would be willing to go into a residential home and that this might be the best thing, as they both get older, in that he would be looked after and she could still visit as often as she liked and could take him out. 7

The outcome is possibly that she will pay lip service to this and just continue to manipulate the situation to her own misguided satisfaction and Thomas will probably regress with the cycle of events recurring. $\frac{3}{12}$

Commentary

In the initial question about Thomas, confidentiality and the GP's responsibility to his patients is tested. The importance of forward planning is also reflected in the answers. The candidate's management skills are tested on the second page and to score top marks (14%) the ability to give the physical, social and psychological aspects shows that the examiner wishes the candidate to consider the problem in its entirety.

Question 17.3 deals with Thomas after his discharge from hospital and tests the doctor's attitudes as well as his attitudes to the patient and his fiancée. On the next page the fiancée who is not your patient takes a more dominant role and the answer deals with the options available at this point. The mark of 14% reflects the importance. The case develops with difficult decisions being needed as to where the patient is to be managed.

The problem ends by considering how Thomas's capabilities should be assessed, looking at his skills for everyday living and how his fiancée fits into his management. This is followed by communication about the case conference and the fiancée's likely reaction to this. Twenty-four per cent of the marks are given for the last two pages.

Case 18

Answers

Mr Jack is an 88-year-old retired policeman who lives with his 90-year-old wife in a modern local authority house, 2½ miles from your surgery. He has a history of chronic obstructive airways disease and a previous myocardial infarction. His wife is not on your NHS list. They tend to be very independent. They have no family.

18.1 What problems are likely to arise as they get older?

Problems of elderly patients living at a distance from the
    surgery.
  Likelihood of increased requests for home visits, 'after hours
    calls'.   2
Problems of separate doctors.
  No knowledge of Mrs Jack's medical history.
  Limitations on amount of medical intervention one can give
    to the couple.   2
Effect of past medical history on needs of health care (relative
    to Mr Jack).
  increasing disability
    congestive cardiac failure
    further myocardial infarction
    cerebral anoxia
  decreasing mobility
    affecting independence.   4
Effect of age on ability to cope with health and remain in the
    community.
  greater dependence on community aid
  clash with independence
  more frequent house calls
  compliance with medication
  risk of polypharmacy
  difficulties if either require hospitalization
  planned need (or persuasion) for residential or supervised
    care
  how much one can intervene with patient's preferred
    independence.   8
                                —
                               16

You are asked to visit Mr Jack at home because of an exacerbation of his chest condition. He tells you he has got dirty spit, and is having difficulty breathing. He has a fever, is obviously dyspnoeic, and has sounds in his chest compatible with a super-imposed chest infection. His wife is hobbling around on a Zimmer, and very anxious.

18.2 Detail factors which would influence your decision whether to treat him at home or admit him.

Clinical assessment
   Is he ill enough to be admitted
   Previous knowledge of how patient reacts to illness.   4
Standard of care at home
   Ability of wife to look after him
   How often can GP visit
   Acceptance of nurse; home help; health visitor
   Ability to obtain and comply with medication
   Standard of nourishment.   6
Social Factors
   Old couple
   Living on own
   Facilities within the house
   Ease of access to toilet
   Proximity of shops, and chemist.   4
Likely effect of hospitalization
   Separation of couple
   Loneliness of partners
   Risk of rapid institutionalization. $\frac{2}{16}$

You reluctantly accept his plea that he is not bad enough for hospital, but when your assistant visits two days later, he is confronted by a neighbour who says Mr Jack ought to be in hospital and Mrs Jack cannot cope.

Your assistant manages to placate the neighbour, and comes to discuss the situation with you, having said he would have an answer tomorrow.

18.3 What do you and your assistant discuss?

Effect of assistant visiting rather than known practitioner
   feeling of '2nd class' treatment.   2

Review of the case to date
    initial 'persuasion' to keep him at home
    any alterations in physical condition in last 2 days
    deterioration
    improvement.   3
Attitude of neighbour
    initially may have been willing to help
    has the burden and responsibility become too much?
    may have additional information which the couple have
        withheld not to upset the doctor.   4
Is admission now indicated
    better clinically for Mr Jack
    effect of separation of the couple
    will wife cope?   2
Contact with wife's GP
    will he be interested in helping? $\underline{1}$
                $\overline{12}$

Having decided that admission would be appropriate, your assistant telephones the hospital, and is told that there won't be a bed for at least 2 days in Mr Jack's usual respiratory unit.

18.4 What can be done at this stage?

Decision to be made
    Wait for the bed: explain to couple and neighbour
    Offer service of nurse, home help, voluntary body (may be
        refused by patient)
    Risk of something happening while waiting and legal
        implications
    Admit elsewhere as emergency with explanation
    May not be welcome to patient or other unit   6
Domiciliary Visit by consultant of usual unit
    Appropriate use of this service for second opinion to back up
        your management and placate neighbour
    Inappropriate if used just to force an admission   3
Discuss with Mrs Jack's GP
    If she is to be left at home
    Advantage of waiting for the bed to allow arrangements to
        be made for her $\underline{1}$
                $\overline{10}$

After his discharge from hospital, you find Mr Jack alone in the house. His wife was admitted to a local authority home while he was in hospital, but was admitted from there to the local geriatric hospital as an emergency. Mr Jack is very aggrieved at his wife's 'mis-management', and says her doctor should be struck off, as he had obviously been mis-managing her.

18.5 How do you react to this, and discuss his immediate management?

Necessity to rapidly defuse a potentially dangerous situation.
 attempt to keep him calm
 quietly ask what happened to his wife
 find out from the hospital
 ethical problem
 find out from her doctor.   4
Assessment of immediate needs when he is on his own.
 can he cope: make food etc.
 compliance with therapy
 supervision
  nurse
  neighbour: has she had enough?
  home help: will he have one?
  social worker
  frequent follow-up visit by doctor. $\frac{6}{10}$

On your next visit, Mr Jack produces Mrs Jack's medical card, and says he wants you to take her on your list. He has signed the card.

18.6 What options are open to you?

Attempt to find out if Mrs Jack really wants to change doctor.
 See her herself in hospital
 Contact her own practitioner if on good terms with him
 Ideally she should have signed the card but most areas
  accept an 'on behalf of' signature.   5
May have to explain the procedure for change.
 May not be possible immediately
 No problem if a 'change of address'
 If same address; both doctors to sign, or by giving notice to
  the health board. $\frac{3}{8}$

You accept the wife on your list. She comes home from the hospital. You find she was admitted to the geriatric department because of dehydration, and failure to eat in the local authority home. There is also a diagnosis of sideroblastic anaemia and osteoarthritis. A referral has been made to orthopaedics for consideration of right hip replacement, and the orthopaedic surgeons have agreed to do this. Mr Jack says something will have to be done also about his wife's eyesight. The hospital told them she had a cataract.

18.7 How do you feel about the management of Mrs Jack now, and what steps would you take?

Exploration of causes of sideroblastic anaemia and original
    failure to eat and dehydration.
  neoplasm
  senile or toxic dementia
  depression
  loneliness and sadness
  iatrogenic—inappropriate therapy.   5
Assess implications of hip replacement in an already frail 90
    year old.
  trauma of operation and anaesthetic
  post operative complications
  is it really indicated
  possibility of a planned admission so that Mr Jack can be
    cared for.   8
Assess visual problem.
  confirm the diagnosis
  priority in relation to hip problem
  effect on her in the house
  effect on her mobility.   2
Can referral wait.
  problem of referral to two clinics simultaneously.   1
                                          16

The Jacks settle down with Mrs Jack waiting for her hip replacement and in the interval she has had one cataract attended to. All has settled down quite well until one evening when you are called to Mrs Jack who is in congestive heart failure, and has to be admitted as an emergency. Mr Jack remains at home, and the next morning when discussing the couple with your health visitor and nurse, your receptionist informs you that a neighbour of Mr Jack has just 'phoned to say that he has been coughing up blood all night and that something will have to be done for him.

18.8 What do you do?

Arrange to visit as soon as possible yourself.	2
Assess clinically.	
exacerbation of chronic obstructive airways disease	
congestive cardiac failure	
embolus	
bronchial carcinoma.	2
Assess if admission is again indicated especially in view of:	
Mrs Jack being in hospital	
recent admission of Mr Jack	
his possible inability to cope	
possible reluctance of neighbour to help with the primary	
care team.	4
Formulate a plan of action for the couple to attempt to avoid	
even further breakdown.	
becoming unable to remain in the community	
may be difficult to persuade them to accept this	
include the neighbour in the general discussion to let her see	
that something is being done.	4
	12

Commentary

The MEQ about the Jacks begins by considering the problems of ageing and the demands this makes on the GP. Question 18.2 presents the problem of where this age group should be managed. The elderly take up a considerable proportion of the GP's time and this is reflected with two higher levels of capitation fee for the over 65's and over 75's. This importance is also considered by the examiner who awards 32% for the first two questions.

In the third question the examiner gives 4% for the neighbour's attitude, not surprising since she will play an important part in the elderly couple's management. In question 18.5 the candidate's attitudes both to his patient and his colleagues are being tested and on the following page decision making after considering a range of options.

Knowledge and skills in managing multiple pathology is tested in question 18.7 with a mark of 16% reflecting its importance for the general practitioner.

Case 19

Answers

Tom and Jessie Scott, although your patients for many years, are rarely seen in the surgery. Tom, 50, is a miner whilst Jessie works part-time as a secretary for the NCB. They have a son Bill, who is 25 and has followed his father into the mines. The local papers are full of the possibility of a mining strike, when Tom presents himself at your surgery. He complains of severe gripping chest pains, which spread to his left arm and seem to be associated with exertion.

19.1 What is your differential diagnosis at this stage?

Angina
Oesophageal
Cervical spine
Psychological
Malingering
Malignancy
Trauma   3

19.2 Outline your management of Tom at this consultation.

Clear history of pain
Smoking, drinking history
Family history of ischaemic heart disease, hypertension,
    diabetes mellitus
Current stresses   3
Tom's feeling *re*: pain   2
Examination including cardiovascular, neck movements,
    respiratory system, muscle tenderness, signs of increased
    lipids   1
Explanation to Tom   1
Consider base line investigation (FBC, chest X-ray, electro-
    cardiogram, lipids, urine)   1
Arrange certification   1
Education *re*: diet and smoking   1
Drug therapy: glyceryl trinitrate with or without beta blocker
    or calcium antagonist   1
Consider hospital if severe pain or increasing frequency.   1
                                                                  ――
                                                                   15

Tom is a heavy smoker, forty a day. As is the local custom he drinks
large volumes of beer at weekends, but none during the week. From
your history and examination you believe he may have developed
angina. In view of his employment you decide to certify him unfit
for work.

19.3 What do you say to Tom?

Explanation in words he will understand, covering life style/
    smoking   3
Need to rest from work till stable
Simple explanation of angina
Offer a chance to be questioned
Explanation aims of therapy   3

**19.4 Outline the short and long term consequences of this
diagnosis for Tom.**

Short Term
    Tom's anger
    Disbelief
    Reluctance to change   3
Long Term
    Change of employment
    Possible financial hardship   2
    Change of role in family
    Change of role in peer group   3
    Medical deterioration
        e.g. bypass or heart failure.

                                                 1

Four weeks later when the strike has become a reality, you are called
to see Tom at home. You had prescribed glyceryl trinitrate and beta
blockers to control his angina and initially this seemed to be
successful. When you see him he is still complaining of chest pain on
exertion and he looks flat and apathetic. While you are in his home
you notice that Jessie has taken on a new lease of life and seems a
much more outgoing woman than you remember.

19.5 Why might Tom's angina not be improving?

Poor compliance
Rejection of diagnosis
Inability to afford drugs

Wrong initial diagnosis	1
Angina deterioration despite therapy	1
Depression	1

**19.6 Give reasons for Tom and Jessie's apparent incon-
　　　gruities and any long term consequences you can forsee.**

Tom a 'male', now dependent.	3
Jessie	
Rediscovery of mother role?	
Now major bread winner	
? outside interests e.g. other man	
Local support group?	
? more money for home rather than alcohol.	3
Consequences	
Possible marital problems if return to normal roles	
Depression in Tom	
Increased drinking in Tom.	$\frac{3}{15}$

Tom tells you that he is being called a 'scab' by his workmates, who
believe he is fabricating his symptoms to avoid picket duty. He tells
you that he wants to be 'signed off' for the next week.

19.7 Outline your response to Tom.

Display empathy	2
Reassure that condition is genuine	1
Explain danger of picket line	
stress	
physical exertion	
violence	3
Explain unhappy about 'signing off'	1
Offer to speak to Union if will help.	$\frac{1}{8}$

Tom decides to join the strike despite your advice. Three days later
you are called to see him at home late at night. Jessie tells you that he
has been in police custody for a few hours charged with assaulting a
Police Officer whilst on picket duty. Jessie is extremely upset and

crying. Concerned neighbours are pressing you to 'give her something'.

19.8 What problems do you face at this time, and how could you deal with them?

Possible anger as your advice disregarded	1
Emotional upset of Tom and wife may exacerbate angina	1
Pressure to prescribe from neighbours	2
Possible legal involvement	1
Danger of being seen to take sides in small community.	1
Options	
Attempt to clear room of neighbours	
Talk to Jennie. Allow her to voice her anger	3
Consider role of short term tranquillizer	
Recognize short term gain of tranquillizer	2
Assess Tom's state	
? angina	
? injury	2
If injury or serious exacerbation of angina, consider hospital	1
Arrange follow-up for both.	1
	15

You spend some time talking to Jessie who settles down. Tom tells you that he was merely part of the crowd when arrested. He asks if he should get a solicitor to fight his case and also asks if you would provide him with medical evidence as to his innocence.

19.9 How would you respond to these two requests, and why?

Agree needs legal help	1
? involve Union	1
Explain unable to give medical evidence	1
Do not reject him	1
Avoid unnatural hopes being built up	1
Offer to speak to solicitor if helps.	1
	6

As you are leaving the house Bill angrily tells you that he is sick of having no money and that he is having to sell his own home as he can no longer afford to pay the mortgage. All this is going to change he says as he is going to do 'a bit of thieving'.

19.10 What problems do you face, and how would you manage them?

Confidentially	2
Responsibility to community as a whole	1
Responsibility to patient	1
Responsibility to family if caught.	1
Actions:	
Advise against	2
Outline dangers in short term and long term for himself and family	2
Offer health visitor or social worker help to clarify financial state.	2
Consider support from:	
Union	
Local support group.	3
	14

While discussing this case with your partners the next day, your senior partner declares that the strike is causing a terrible increase in work. Your other partners nod in agreement. You are, however, uncertain about this.

19.11 How could you confirm or deny your partner's statement?

Use ancillary staff to collect simple workload figures using:	3
Appointment book	
House call book	
Night visit claims	4
Base pre-strike sample on similar time of year	
Attempt to have same variables	
e.g. partner holidays	
epidemics	
health scares	3
If diagnostic registration carried out	
classify contacts by diagnostic group.	3
	13

Commentary

When Tom presents in the first question with chest pain the examiner only awards three marks for the differential diagnosis but twelve marks for a comprehensive management play. In question 19.3 the importance of communication is demonstrated and six marks are given for what the doctor says to Tom.

The importance of psychology is demonstrated after this when Tom and Jessie behave differently: an understanding of this behaviour scores 9%. In question 19.8 when Jessie is upset decision making is tested: the candidate has to mention his options and make the appropriate choice. This is an important area of assessment in the MEQ with this being reflected in the examiner's scoring of 15%.

Statements about workload are often made without any evidence: the final page deals with collecting evidence on this topic.

Case 20

Answers

You are called late one night to see a febrile two-year-old girl. The family are new to your list and you have no records available.

20.1 Which areas would you cover in this consultation?

History of presenting problem	
Past medical history of child	
Recent past medical history of other children	3
Recent past medical history of family	
Social history of family, local contacts	
Parents employment	3
Drugs being taken	3
Allergy	
Relevant physical examination	1
Explanation of findings	2
Relevant therapy	1
Review appointment	1
	14

You discover that Tom and Jennie have moved into the area whilst Tom, who is unskilled, looks for work. They have two children, Fergus who is seven and Fiona who is two. The family have no relatives in the area and have been housed by the council on an estate usually used for 'problem families'.

20.2 What problems might this family face?

Lack of support from family or neighbours	3
Poor quality housing	
Poor quality neighbours	
Stigma of address	
Financial hardship	
Indifference from professional agencies	
Inability of agencies to help with problems	3

Increased incidence of minor illness
Increased dependence on medical service
Increased risk of anxiety/depression
Increased risk of marital disharmony
Increased risk of childhood behaviour problems 　　　　　3

20.3 Are there any ways that you can help them?

Development of doctor/patient relationship
Reasonable availability of doctor 　　　　　　　　　　　　　2
Education *re*: availability of health visitor and social worker
Education *re*: local pressure groups
Education *re*: arrangements for appointments and house calls　3
Training of reception staff in attitudes to deprived
Development of health education e.g. contraception or minor
　　illness care. 　　　　　　　　　　　　　　　　　　　　　$\frac{1}{15}$

Fiona has a self-limiting upper respiratory tract infection which you treat conservatively. You lose sight of the family until you are approached by your Health Visitor one month later. She tells you that she is concerned because Fiona is 'failing to thrive'. She has asked for the mother and child to attend your surgery later that day.

20.4 What is meant by 'failing to thrive'? How would you confirm this at your initial consultation?

Definition. Recognizing inadequate weight gain relative to age
　　and height. 　　　　　　　　　　　　　　　　　　　　　3
Percentile charts.
Child below third centile. 　　　　　　　　　　　　　　　　3

20.5 If the child is failing to thrive, list likely reasons why, and how you would initially investigate these possibilities as a General Practitioner.

Causes
　　Familial
　　Diet
　　Emotional deprivation
　　Chronic illness e.g. asthma, coronary heart disease, renal
　　　　disease or urinary tract infection
　　Malabsorption e.g. coeliac, fibrocystic. 　　　　　　　　3

Examine:
   Clinical history and parents' height
   Simple dietary history
   Clinical history. Input from health visitor. Exam ? bruises
   History. Examination of relevant system
   Peak expiratory flow. Urinalysis and culture
   History. Stool exam
   Consider referral for sweat test   3
   Consider paediatric referral in absence of obvious cause
   Ensure percentile chart in record
   Ensure health visitor follow-up.   3
                                                                 ──
                                                                 15

You discover that Fiona eats an extremely deficient diet. This appears to be made up of packet soups and crisps. Jennie seems totally unconcerned by this diet.

20.6 Give reasons for Jennie's attitude.

Mother's dietary ignorance   2
Poor mother/child bonding   1
Finances demand poor diet   2
   ? power off
   ? alcohol and cigarettes
Mother's depression   1
Housing with inadequate kitchen.   1

20.7 How would you manage this situation?

Discover mother's view   1
Educate mother by self, health visitor, dietitian   1
Educate that love requires nutrition   1
Consider: is child 'at risk'? Involve social services   2
Involve social services to ensure allowances claimed   1
Consider drug therapy if mother depressed   1
Consider pressure on housing department.   1
                                                                 ──
                                                                 15

Your Health Visitor agrees to monitor the family closely and the Social Services become involved to ensure adequate finance for the family. You are approached by the Social Worker who asks if she can give the family's name to a local group who provide holidays and toys for needy families.

20.8 How would you respond to this, and why?

Recognize place of confidentiality

Social worker or GP must discuss this with family first

Recognize danger of 'charity' label

Care not to damage doctor/social worker relationship by recognizing the caring nature of social worker request.

Jennie is obviously pleased by your interest in the family and tells you with great embarrassment one day that Fergus still wets the bed.

20.9 What are the possible causes for this?

Failure to develop bladder control (recognize high percentage at this age)

Emotional factors e.g. home, school, sibs, other children

Urinary tract infection

Domestic problems e.g. out of order toilet, smell, out of door toilet

Metabolic, neurological, mental retardation (rare).

Jennie agrees to bring Fergus to see you and when you examine him he seems to have no physical abnormality.

20.10 List possible management options and their pros and cons.

All   Discover if any previous treatment

Urine culture. Urinalysis—refer if abnormality

Options

No therapy.

Accept a variation on normal, time will cure

Pros   Develops understanding of problem

Avoid drugs and therapy failure

Cons May be unacceptable to family

No initial obvious help

Star chart and limit late fluids.

Pros Cheap
Simple
Involves family

Cons Relapse rate
Understanding of positive attitude to success rather
than failure required   3

Pad and Bell

Pros Active
Avoid drugs
Involves child

Cons May disturb the whole family
Availability of equipment   3

Tricyclics at night.

Pros Effective

Cons Dangerous drugs in house
Relapse rate
Side effects $\dfrac{3}{15}$

_____

Sitting thinking about this case makes you recognize that there are deficiencies in your practice organization.

20.11 How can a GP organize his practice to maximize the help he gives to socially deprived patients?

Recognition of at-risk groups
Good records
At risk registers   3
Team approach. Involve health visitor, social worker, district nurse
Team communication   3
Practice policy e.g. receptionist education
Doctor's management of problems   3
Recognition of areas of responsibility of different team members
Develop relationships with voluntary agencies, self help groups, housing department.   3

    $\overline{12}$

Commentary

The MEQ about Tom and Jenny commences with an important
problem in general practice: a family presenting and there are no
records available. This family have just moved to a problem housing
scheme adding a further dimension. An understanding of this
situation in the first three questions is rewarded by the examiner
and 29% is awarded. High marks are awarded (7%) later for suggesting reasons for the mother's lack of concern about Fiona's diet
with 8% being given for the management of this situation.

   In question 20.10 the candidate is asked to work out a management plan for enuresis: this tests his problem solving ability, his
range of alternatives with the implications of each choice. The
problem ends by testing the candidate's knowledge of socially
deprived patients, an important problem especially in the Inner
Cities.